Praise for *Health: Spirit, Country and Culture* ...

'Aboriginal and Torres Strait Islanders have developed the longest and richest continuous culture on earth. They have done this through their profound understanding of what it means to be healthy – as an individual, as a family, as a community and for Country, and that is the focus of this wonderful book. Written by Professors Shawana Andrews, Sandra Eades, Fiona Stanley, who bring together what it has meant to be healthy in the past, how to apply that knowledge today and what it can tell us about navigating the health challenges that will confront us all in the future.'

—Dr Doug Hilton, AO, FAA, FTSE, FAHMS,
CSIRO Chief Executive

'An exceptional book authored by three highly respected researchers in the health space. It offers a profound exploration of the lived experiences and unique Indigenous perspectives on the history and challenges of health for Indigenous peoples. The inclusion of planetary health was an unexpected but welcome addition, enhancing the depth of this book.'

—Professor Kelvin Kong

'*Health* describes the powerful and effective Indigenous knowledges for our health and wellbeing, and it is so much more than you might expect from a Western perspective – in these pages are Aboriginal ways of knowing, being and doing with a common theme: the importance of building relationships.'

—Thomas Mayo

'This important book brings together what counts in First Nations' health by people who know. It shows there is no mystery about the solutions for First Nations people's health and wellbeing. What's needed is the grit and determination by th strings to listen and act.'

—Dr Norman Swan, AM, FAHMS

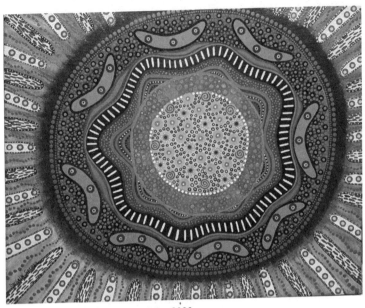

Danielle Gorogo, *Sharing Knowledge*, 2023

'Caring and sharing through, with, and for the community, our children, our Elders and ourselves is important for us as a collective culture. Reinforcing the strength and resilience of our culture can be gained from extended family networks and communities. Our connection is maintained through respective knowledge and actions to share and care for each other and for Country.'
—Danielle Gorogo

Danielle Gorogo is a Clarence Valley First Nations artist living in the Northern Rivers region, NSW. She is a direct descendent of the Dunghutti, Gumbaynggirr and Bundjalung nations. Danielle's multifaceted cultural heritage, which includes First Nations Australian, Papua New Guinean, Māori and Micronesian ancestry, is reflected in her art.

HEALTH

Aboriginal and Torres Strait Islander peoples are advised that this book contains the names of people who have passed away.

HEALTH

Spirit, Country and Culture

SHAWANA ANDREWS,
SANDRA EADES &
FIONA STANLEY

First published in Australia in 2024 by Thames & Hudson Australia
Wurundjeri Country, 132A Gwynne Street, Cremorne, Victoria 3121

Health © Thames & Hudson Australia 2024

Introduction © Margo Ngawa Neale 2024
Text © Shawana Andrews, Sandra Eades & Fiona Stanley 2024

Text on pp. 137–8 references Adam Brumm's, '"The Falling Sky": Symbolic and Cosmological Associations of the Mt William Greenstone Axe Quarry, Central Victoria, Australia', *Cambridge Archaeological Journal*, Cambridge University Press, 20(2), pp. 179–96, 2010 © Cambridge University Press, reproduced with permission.

Copyright in all texts, artworks and images is held by the creators or their representatives, unless otherwise stated.

Thames & Hudson Australia thanks those who have generously given permission for their works to be quoted in this book.

27 26 25 24   5 4 3 2 1

The moral right of the authors has been asserted.

All rights reserved. No part of this publication may be reproduced or transmitted in any form or by any means, electronic or mechanical, including photocopy, recording or any other information storage or retrieval system, without prior permission in writing from the publisher.

ISBN 978-1-760-76340-4 (paperback)
ISBN 978-1-760-76341-1 (ebook)

 A catalogue record for this book is available from the National Library of Australia

Every effort has been made to trace accurate ownership of copyrighted text and visual materials used in this book. Errors or omissions will be corrected in subsequent editions, provided notification is sent to the publisher.

  This project has been assisted by the Australian Government through the Australia Council, its arts funding and advisory body.

Front cover: *Sharing Knowledge* by Danielle Gorogo

Series editor: Margo Ngawa Neale
Cover design: Nada Backovic
Typesetting: Megan Ellis
Project editor: Bernadette Foley
Editors: Bernadette Foley and Marg Bowman
Assistant editor: Bridget Caldwell-Bright

Printed and bound in Australia by McPherson's Printing Group

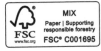 FSC® is dedicated to the promotion of responsible forest management worldwide. This book is made of material from FSC®-certified forests and other controlled sources.

Thames & Hudson Australia wishes to acknowledge that Aboriginal and Torres Strait Islander peoples are the first storytellers of this nation and the Traditional Custodians of the land on which we live and work. We acknowledge their continuing culture and pay respect to Elders past and present.

thamesandhudson.com.au

It is with deep respect that we dedicate this book to Dr Yunupiŋu of the Gumatj clan and Dr Lowitja O'Donoghue, a Yankunytjatjara woman. Both were outstanding leaders in health and political activism. They challenged the overwhelming colonial ways of doing, and pushed self-determining agendas that empowered culture, Country, identity and language – all of which constitute Aboriginal health and wellbeing.

Dr Yunupiŋu, born 30 June 1948 and died 3 April 2023.
Dr Lowitja O'Donoghue, born 1 August 1932 and
died 4 February 2024.

NOTE ON STYLE AND SPELLING

The First Knowledges series seeks to honour the individual voices and stylistic preferences of each book's authors. Readers may also note that for different language groups, variant spellings occur for similar words, cultural groups or names.

NOTE ABOUT AUSTRALIAN NATIVE MEDICINES

You may expect that this book would include information about the vast knowledge of using native plants for medicinal treatments. We recognise that there is widespread and increasing interest in Australian native foods and medicines. However, it would have been impossible for us to write about them all, as they differ so much across the continent, with considerable variations in plants and environments. Vivienne Hansen, a Noongar Elder, and John Horsfall have published two books on these knowledges for the southwest corner of Western Australia alone, and Madison King and John Horsfall have published a book about the medicinal plants of the Kimberley region (*see* 'Further reading'). If we had chosen the Noongar or the Kimberley information, it would have meant excluding all the other regions with their well-known foods and medicines. Also, there is increasing concern among Aboriginal people about the intellectual property of this information and we were keen not to breach any legal or cultural laws. We have mentioned some Australian native foods and medicines in the book in relation to aspects of Aboriginal life but have not given detailed information.

CONTENTS

First Knowledges: An Introduction *Margo Ngawa Neale*		1
1	Personal perspectives *Shawana Andrews, Sandra Eades & Fiona Stanley*	15
2	Place, relationships and futures *Shawana Andrews*	34
3	Birthing on Country and dying on Country *Fiona Stanley*	49
4	Community control and primary health care *Sandra Eades*	73
5	Indigenous people and hospital care *Shawana Andrews*	90
6	Traditional life for health *Sandra Eades*	108
7	Health and cultural practice *Shawana Andrews*	123
8	Aboriginal worldviews in mainstream services *Fiona Stanley*	139
9	An Indigenous-led health research agenda *Sandra Eades & Fiona Stanley*	157
10	Planetary health: Ancient wisdom for modern problems *Fiona Stanley, Sandra Eades & Shawana Andrews*	175
Uluru Statement from the Heart: What it means for First Knowledges – Health		187
Acknowledgements		190
Image credits		193
Notes		195
Further reading		210
Index		213
About the authors		226

FIRST KNOWLEDGES

MARGO NGAWA NEALE, SERIES EDITOR

Country is the DNA of the First Knowledges series. It is the link that binds all books in the series, just as it connects all First Peoples. Our knowledge system is drafted by Country. Our lives are governed by Country. Country holds the knowledge that enabled us to survive and thrive over the past 65 millennia. It governs us, teaches us, nurtures us and heals us. It is our raison d'être.

This is the eighth book in the First Knowledges series. *Health: Spirit, Country and Culture* demonstrates how the Western system of health care has attempted to erase what went before, in this area as in all areas, and to superimpose a system that contravenes the laws of the land and her people, supplanting spirit and culture with drugs, pills, doctors and interventionist procedures. The authors propose the marriage of the two systems as the only way forward.

In chapter 2, Shawana Andrews writes: 'Prior to colonisation, health was not something to be sought and attained.' It occurred naturally because of the lifestyle, and along with diet, it was inextricably connected to Country. As the authors say, it was built on a deep knowledge of environments, seasons, sustainable harvesting practices, processing techniques and nutritional values. Food security and nutrition did not exist in isolation but were embedded in a complex structure of relationships.

Still today, food production is linked to the sustainability of Country and is supported through kinship and totemic systems, which nourish the mind and spirit every minute of life and indeed death. Death is conceived as the reverse process, a stage of life rather than an event defined in time and place: 'a gentle leaching of the body and spirit back into the earth'.[1] Smoking and cleansing ceremonies are carried out to ensure that the spirit does not come back and become a discontented soul lurking in the bush and waterways, threatening harm to the community. It focuses on prevention, not cure, and treats the whole person, as the book's subtitle reads: *Spirit, Country and Culture*. Aboriginal health involves a holistic rather than a unitary view where the body is treated separately from spirit, mind and Country.

Country provides medicine we now call bush medicine, which has become an industry in itself. Many ingredients have found their way into Western pharmaceuticals. On one hand this is an example of the partnering of the Western and Indigenous systems. At the same time, the appropriation of Indigenous knowledges is becoming a serious issue in the domains of intellectual property rights, recognition and recompense.

Country also provides several multi-functional medicinal elements, such as a range of clays that are used as pigments for painting and other uses. Kaolin, for example, is a white clay used as an effective binding treatment for diarrhoea and as paint for body painting and other ceremonial markings. Red ochre is regarded by many as the blood of the ancestors, and when mixed with water, saliva, animal fat, oil or blood, is used for both ceremonial and functional purposes. It was applied to rock, weapons, ceremonial objects, skin and hair. It is also used for the care of wounds such as burns, sores and insect bites, and as protection from the weather. When mixed with other medicinal substances such as sap, leaves, ashes or oil it can be applied to the skin. Ochre's rich iron compounds and mineral content have antiseptic and styptic properties.

I recall experiences from my years living in the camps and outstations of Arnhem Land during the Homelands movement of the 1970s, crushing green ants and mixing them with water to gargle for a sore throat. As an antiseptic, it is rich in formic acid used in pharmaceutical gargle solutions. For back aches, sore muscles, flu and colds I would take a bush sauna. This entailed lying in a pit that had warm rocks covered by a layer of eucalyptus leaves moistened with water to create steam. I was then blanketed with another layer of warm eucalyptus leaves and water, followed by a topping of paper bark that was used like alfoil to keep the steam in. It was like being cooked in a Māori hangi with the temperature adjusted.

Exercise was built naturally into the lifestyle at the camps and outstations. With only your own legs to get you around and no one-stop shop, such as a supermarket to supply your food and personal needs, and no electricity and running water, one had to be on the move all day. I personally can attest to this. To do something as simple as making myself a cup of tea in the camp involved a long, hot and dusty walk to the river. Then I had to light a fire, often with damp wood, dole out the mugs of tea to our seniors first and if I was lucky I might get half a cup at best until I did it again. This happened a couple of times a day. Camps were always located some distance from the river and surrounding bush, which was cleared for some 20 or 30 metres for fear of malevolent spirits. We lived in gunyahs in a hot dust bowl several hundred metres from the river.

Mental health was assured in traditional times by living a life of stability and certainty; a lifestyle that has been ruptured through colonisation. As we know, the Western system fails those who fall between the cracks. Where the traditional kinship system applies, everyone has a valued place, which is predetermined and endows a person from birth with a sense of belonging and purpose. Through the sophisticated skin group system, your relationship to every element of nature, both animate and inanimate, and every person, past, present and not yet born, is preordained. Roles and responsibilities are defined, and you have many family members throughout your community, beyond the biological family, who are responsible for your upbringing. These days this would be called the logical family. It conforms to logic rather convention.

Cultural principles remain to a large extent even in the more urbanised parts of the country and are being strengthened progressively through reclamation and revitalisation. Incompatibility with institutions such as hospitals and other Western medical practices is not hard to understand. If a person is hospitalised, for example, several other kinship relatives, who may not be biologically related, must be there as well. Who signs the consent forms? Convention dictates a biological relative, but through the kinship system people can have familial relationships – such as parents, siblings or aunts – without being biologically related.

If 'sorry business' held after the death of a person is in progress for a senior person, then the patient must leave hospital to attend, even if it's against the doctor's orders. Actions like this are sometimes viewed by the hospital as being irresponsible, disobedient, useless, or subject to other racist judgements, unless there are Aboriginal health workers on-site who have some understanding of the protocols and obligations. Then they could reach a compromise. As a case in point, the authors describe a patient from the Royal Melbourne Hospital with a serious respiratory condition who was 'allowed' to go back to Country to die. This hospital understood the cultural necessity and provided a small generator to run the respirator. In most cases it is ignorance rather than an intention to be disrespectful, as exemplified by one example in the book when a well-meaning doctor asked an Aboriginal patient if ATSI (which stands for Aboriginal and Torres Strait Islander) was a disease.

If Country is healthy, people are healthy. Conversely if Country is sick, people are sick. Aboriginal people kept this Country sustainable and healthy for more than 65,000 years, yet in the past 232 years since the arrival of people not from this country, the country has become progressively unhealthy to the point of crisis. People are becoming progressively sicker as we lurch from one environmental and climatic disaster to another.

Though hard to believe, even Lieutenant James Cook understood the centrality of Country to Aboriginal people's lives. He wrote in his journal on 23 August 1770: 'they may appear to some to be the most wretched people upon Earth, but they are far happier than we Europeans; being wholy [*sic*] unacquainted not only with the superfluous but the necessary conveniencies [*sic*] so much sought after in Europe, they are happy in not knowing the use of them at all'. He further noted the people's tranquillity, equality and lack of need of material possessions such as houses and clothes, acknowledging that Country provides for all.

We can no longer ignore Indigenous values and practices. In chapter 10 of this book we read that 'Planetary health has now become an emerging Western concept that *at last* acknowledges that human health is intricately connected to the health of natural systems within the Earth's biosphere and that the health of all species is deeply reliant on it'.[2] The authors refer to 'the marriage of revitalised Aboriginal knowledges with the necessary Western medicine to manage the diseases that First Nations people have faced since colonisation'. It is not surprising then, that this call-to-action has become a plea from authors of the other books in the series. Marcia Langton and Aaron Corn in *Law: The Way of the Ancestors* write about how the two systems of law must find a way of working together, while in *Astronomy* the authors write about how Indigenous astronomy can complement Western astronomy. In fact, this need for the meeting of the two ways was one of the prime instigators for the series. I would maintain that the world has woken up to this truth with a sudden jerk in the last five years or so. This would account for the great take up of this series by readers across the spectrum. The moons are lined up.

As you will read in chapter 2, 'Western health systems are comparatively new and are largely built on biomedical constructions of health, which are based on the presence or absence of disease, and on reductionist science.'[3] The knowledge of Aboriginal healing, however, has been deepening for as long as Aboriginal people have lived on this continent: if you listen to the creation stories passed down you learn that we were created at the same time as the land. Our system of health and wellbeing evolved around people, Country and culture and not around science. This is not to say there is no science: it is integrated into all fields of knowledge. The Indigenous system does not compartmentalise knowledge into separate disciplines but rather it operates as an integrated whole. Culture can be likened to a master cylinder and Country the archive that stores the knowledges.

How Country and culture work together in an adaptive system of Western medical and Aboriginal thinking is demonstrated in Professor Sandra Eades's story of her mother's last days, where she was surrounded by family at home on Country. As Sandra says, 'we were in control and the cultural aspects of care were intertwined with the need for Western medicines'. At dawn her mother's totem, the culbardi, magpie, attended her passing, signifying that Country was calling for her to rejoin the ancestors. In another case, an Aboriginal woman had to stay in the Royal Melbourne Hospital, which was distant from Country. So Country was brought to her in the form of earth, which accompanied her burial. There is an increasing number of hospitals with crying rooms or First Nation support rooms for family and community who must be with an ailing or dying person. 'I feel safe, I can cry here,' one of the Elders said, which was a measure of relationship and trust.

Possum skin cloaks have a role in healing in some hospitals, as have other objects that hold the spirit of ancestors' healing power. Many traditional healers, known as the Ngangkari in Central

Australia, have roles in some hospitals to complement the Western roles of physician, therapist, priest and coroner. Smoking ceremonies and other ways of honouring the sacred indicate a dramatic rebirth of Aboriginal knowledge being used to improve the health and wellbeing of First Nations populations and others too.

The most effective strategy for improvements in all types of health is simple yet powerful – it is the involvement of the patients, their families and communities, and Indigenous health workers. The authors provide impressive evidence-based results of better health outcomes due to Aboriginal-led, culturally adaptive ways of providing care. They discuss how input from the community is paramount to success in Aboriginal community participation research programs. These work from the bottom up and contrast with mainstream research projects where non-Indigenous academic researchers often decide on the ideas and the hypotheses with little input from the community they are researching. Framing research without an understanding of the effects of colonisation and root causes will invariably lead to services that fail and cause further dislocation and loss of self-esteem. A well-known, expensive, punitive and traumatising mainstream service, as many viewed it and experienced it, was the 2007 Northern Territory Emergency Response, known as 'The Intervention', as the authors remind us.

Indigenous data sovereignty is at the centre of the concept of Aboriginal Community Participation Action Research methods. The use of Community Reference Groups for all Aboriginal research is core to ensuring that the best-informed decisions are made. But a lot of yarning must go on to build trust, long before the research questions are developed. In response to two centuries of being treated as ethnographic subjects of study with no voice, the authors call for 'No data or research on us without us', a repurposed slogan coined by disability activists, 'Nothing about us without us', used by other authors in this series and others such as Māori activist Linda Tuhiwai Smith.

Another response was a data collection project run by the Telethon Kids Institute in Western Australia, established by Professor Fiona Stanley over a decade ago. Ninety per cent of Indigenous families across the state participated, which was a record response rate. Aboriginal researchers led the project, without whom the data could not have been collected, analysed or interpreted.

As the authors urge, the key to success is building ancient knowledge systems into contemporary institutions. A highly successful community-controlled organisation, the peak body, the National Aboriginal Community Controlled Health Organisation (NACCHO), now has some 550 affiliated clinics that are accessed by more than half a million visitations each year. They are the largest employer of Aboriginal and Torres Strait Islander people in the country.

Negotiating the constraints of Western systems with professionals who can walk in both worlds is a game-changer. A resurgence of interest in traditional Grandmothers' Way of birthing with professionals (both Indigenous and non-Indigenous) who have the expertise of Western medicine and who can drive the revitalisation of Aboriginal worldviews, is life changing. This is abundantly clear in Birthing-and-Dying-on-Country programs.

The message that birthing and dying are not diseases, but rather just part of the cycle of life, shifts the paradigm. These programs can accommodate situations where many who cannot go back to Country physically, can return spiritually through the application of cultural practices. The programs involve birthing trees and placenta gardens, which connect the new child to Mother Earth and provide therapy for grieving mothers who have lost a child or in cases when the child was removed. The authors provide figures that reveal 'that Birthing on Country services reduce, by 60 per cent, the risk of children being taken into care',[4,5] thus 'affirming the power of culture to enhance the confidence and capacity of families'.

Along with the increase in Aboriginal community-controlled medical services comes the increase in the number of Aboriginal doctors, with statistics that are, proportionately, nearly on par with the number of non-Indigenous doctors. The authors also tell us that Year 12 retention rates are on the increase, with nearly 60 per cent of Aboriginal kids completing Year 12 in 2021, compared to 79 per cent for non-Aboriginal youth. This augurs well, but why don't we hear about these positive findings?

Aboriginal leadership in times of crisis is exemplary and is borne out by the way Aboriginal leaders and community managed the COVID-19 pandemic. Aboriginal people, mostly from remote areas, returned to Country and to nature, and clung together as a community, while the non-Indigenous people were directed to isolate themselves from family and community.

This book, *Health*, like other titles in the series, is written in partnership by authors from both cultures, Indigenous and Western.

Professor Fiona Stanley is the most senior and she has been a mentor and guide to the other writers, Associate Professor Shawana Andrews and Professor Sandra Eades, in Western ways, as they have to her in Aboriginal ways. Fiona was both a mentor and a supervisor of Sandra's PhD. Their journey together started many years earlier when their pathways intersected through the various realms of health and wellbeing, in which they are all involved.

It is fitting that the three writers are women, as women in Aboriginal society are seen as the healers and nurturers, as well as the keepers and holders of knowledge for health and wellbeing, especially as they pertain to women and children.

If you have read any other books in the series you will know that in each one you will encounter aspects of art, ceremony, Law and medicine, for example, in varying degrees. In an integrated knowledge system such subjects are viewed together. For example, culture includes Law, is defined by Law, and culture is practised through art and ceremony, just as this book, *Health*, discusses plants, ceremony and art. After all there can be no remedy in the Western medicine toolbox that can address trauma as effectively as can ceremony and ritual, which are an expression of the arts, or at least are expressed in the visual mode of what Westerners call art. So, the recurrence of certain topics across the series is not repetition, but reinforcement and the deepening of knowledge in the way of the Indigenous knowledge system and modes of learning.

We planned for this series to consist of six volumes but the demand for them has been overwhelming. We are now up to eight titles. The world hungers for Indigenous knowledges and has come to the timely realisation that solutions can be found in the ancient system of environmental care. There is such despair at where the capitalist colonialist regime of thinking has led us – our planet is now on the brink and we lurch from one environmental disaster to another.

The first book in the series *Songlines: The Power and Promise* lays down the foundational truths of this continent shaped by Country itself. It reveals how Country holds knowledge, what Songlines are and how they work. The second book, *Design: Building on Country* is a fascinating new look at design from an Indigenous perspective. It demonstrates how building on Country in contemporary times can be an extension of Country as it once was. It urges designers and architects to work with nature as a collaborator and not a usurper. The third book in the series *Country: Future Fire, Future Farming* is a timely call-to-action to employ old methods of working with the land and not against it. To 'farm without fences' as Bill Gammage refers to hunting and gathering methods, or mentoring nature for sustainable food production as Bruce Pascoe sees it. And to use only plantings natural to these soils that are not water hungry or do not need pesticides and fertilisers, which kill it. The fourth book, *Astronomy: Sky Country* encapsulates the Indigenous world view in which land, water and sky are all viewed as Country. It notes how colonisation of the skies with thousands of artificial satellites are obstructing our Songlines or sky-stories with light pollution that interferes with the natural habits of wildlife and humans alike.

Plants: Past, Present and Future, the fifth book in the series, celebrates the deep cultural significance of plants, their medicinal, ceremonial and functional values. *Law: The Way of the Ancestors* shows that Law and culture are indivisible. It too is a timely call for Indigenous Law to become an essential part of Australian nationhood, thus offering a social contract for a unified future. Like the book *Songlines*, it is foundational to the other books in the series. *Innovation: Knowledge and Ingenuity* counters the long-held view in some quarters that First Peoples were frozen in the Stone Age and like the native animals, survived by being unchanging and uninventive and living by instinct. It begs the question how could the First Peoples of an 8-million-square-kilometre continent of such topographic diversity, small in number, live here for 65,000 years and not be masters of innovation and invention?

While it is well known that colonialism has had an enormous impact on Indigenous societies, this series reveals the other side of that coin: the significant influences that Aboriginal and Torres Strait Islander cultures are having on Australian society and history, and the enormous contribution our people are making, which mainstream Australia is beginning to embrace.

1

PERSONAL PERSPECTIVES

SHAWANA ANDREWS

Between the ages of three and six, I travelled the country with my parents, who got jobs locally wherever we were. It was the late 1970s and early 80s. My mum is a Pairrebeenne/Trawlwoolway woman who also has Irish heritage and who grew up in Naarm (Melbourne). My dad is an Indian migrant, with some Scottish heritage, from a town called Dhanbad in India. I didn't attend school until we returned to Melbourne after my brother was born in Perth in 1980.

When I was about eight we went to Central Arnhem Land for a few months, visiting my uncle who worked there. We stayed on a cattle station near the Bulman–Weemol Aboriginal community, about 300 kilometres east of Katherine. While there in the dry season, I would go swimming in the water hole with the kids and the aunties. We had a tractor tyre that we'd float on and have hours of fun with it. We'd catch fish or turtle for lunch and cook it on the fire by the water; it would serve as the main meal on those hot days. The men, who mostly worked at the surrounding cattle stations, would sometimes hunt kangaroo and this would be shared around the fire. The pastoral industry is iconic in the Northern Territory and depended on cheap Aboriginal labour for its success.

Surrounded by speakers of local languages and Aboriginal English, I mostly did not know what was being said, but playing with the kids and the fun we had is etched into my memory. One hot day at the station, there was a fire going to burn off some rubbish and the wind picked up. A piece of burning rubbish flew out and landed on me, burning my leg. There was no clinic or medical facility, so cold water and makeshift dressings were the best my parents could do at the time. On another occasion, my brother became unwell and had to see a doctor and so a 600-kilometre round trip to Katherine was needed. At the time I didn't think much about these incidents and wasn't aware of how the community addressed health issues. When we returned home, however, my mum became really ill with something the doctors in Melbourne couldn't identify. It was Strongyloidiasis, a tropical condition associated with poor living conditions. She was hospitalised and finally treated. Seeing her so sick made me think about health, especially in Aboriginal communities, and what helps or hinders it.

For much of the rest of my childhood we lived in the northwestern suburbs of Melbourne, during which time my sisters came along. Each summer we would set out on our camping holiday to the mighty Snowy River on the lands of the Gunaikurnai people. Our holidays were simple: camping in tents, cooking on the fire, looking at the stars and swimming in the river. We went to the same place every year for my entire childhood and continue to go there now. My siblings and I came to know the river well. The waterline would be different every year and there were subtle changes to the vegetation, but the riverbed and the rocks that formed it were unchanging and these became one of us. We longed to be there, to sit on and swim around the familiar rocks; our favourite was called 'flat rock', on which we could sunbake or dive off into the rushing current. We spent hours on that rock and in the water, catching lizards on the bank, watching dragonflies hatch and kingfishers flitting around the river and in and out of their burrows. Sometimes emus would stroll through our camp, and on a more recent trip, we witnessed something we'd never seen before, an eclipse of bogong moths. We roasted and ate the moths just as the Gunaikurnai people did for at least 2000 years.

My time on this Country distinctly shaped how I understand place and Country. My siblings and I now take our children there. We still love it and it speaks to us when we arrive, the rushing sound of the water, the clinking of the rocks and the echoing call of the crow in the valley. The familiar smell of the trees and the red earth when I'm at the river for just a week or so each year makes me think how well you might come to know a living landscape when you live with it for more than a lifetime. What could generations learn? Sadly, the subtle changes we noticed over forty years have culminated in the river being very unwell now. The combined impact of the Snowy Hydro Scheme and the sustained damage of the brumbies and other introduced species in the region have created an environmental disaster. The mountain pygmy possum of the ranges is endangered, which is related to the decline in the bogong moths; the delicate ecosystem is damaged.

———

In 1999 I graduated with a social work degree. It wasn't the type of degree I had expected; in my naivety I had wanted more, more answers and tools for the questions I had about people and their needs. Instead, I got theories I couldn't relate to and unfair critique when I challenged them. I almost left the course midway, but in it I met Noonuccal woman Lisa Bellear, who delivered a guest lecture. She read one of her poems in her presentation and it was at this point that I understood that I could make of this degree what I wanted and challenge the profession from within. I worked for many years in the hospital system, but it wasn't until I did a Master of Public Health that I found the thinking I was looking for. I would later go on to do a PhD, which I hoped would offer something to Aboriginal women and also to the academy, not only by way of challenge but by bringing Aboriginal women's voice and cultural practice to the fore.

As an adult I have travelled to India with my dad on numerous occasions and each time I have come to understand him a little more. In the country of his birth he becomes dynamic, speaking Hindi and reconnecting to the smells, sounds and feel of the place. Memory, food, relationships and ideas about 'home' form the basis of his connection to place. One of the things I noticed on an early trip to India, when I was about nineteen, was the importance of visiting. We were staying with my aunty and every evening before dinner, we'd get ready to head out to visit family and friends in the village. On these visits we would be offered chai and food and stay for a yarn. I learnt a lot about my dad and my extended family and community in India during these visits. I learnt that visiting is a way to think about being present, in relationship, over time. I learnt that it is intentional as a way to connect, and to transfer histories, family stories, values, lessons and ways of life. Visiting invites memory and I could see its importance for my dad, who left India for Australia in 1969. I recently learned of this same practice in Turtle Island (Canada) in Indigenous communities and how visiting is being used as a research methodology. It got me thinking about my own visiting practices in Australia.

I didn't grow up on Country and I don't live there now. As a child I only visited my mother's Country once, when I was about ten, and it had a distinct impact on me. We visited Dalrymple Briggs's house, which at the time was in Latrobe in Trouwerner (Tasmania), and I learnt about my ancestral grandmothers. Dalrymple Briggs was the daughter of Woretemoeteyenner, who was the daughter of Mannalargenna. I remember being shocked at the violence of Tasmania's history, yet entranced by the stories of enduring fortitude, particularly by the grandmothers. Now I visit regularly, and I take my three daughters too. We go every year and celebrate on Country. I make this visiting intentional for us as a family. We meet our extended family and community at Little Musselroe Bay on Tebrakunna Country, and learn our histories, eat traditional foods and connect. I watch my girls when we are there and they become immersed in their visiting; creating, learning and connecting memory in the place their astronomical ancestors walked to via the Milky Way.

Back in Naarm, my grandmother's kitchen table is another visiting centrepiece. Nanny Mary's kitchen table has seen generations of my family grow up around it, drinking tea and eating food made in the humblest of ways. I remember swinging upside down in the old gnarly apricot tree in the backyard with my cousins, eating the fruit and spitting the seeds as far as we could. We'd be called inside for dinner and the kitchen table would seem like it was heaving with food. In her poem 'Perhaps the World Ends Here', US Poet Laureate Joy Harjo of Muscogee (Creek) Nation writes about the centrality of the kitchen table and its role in hosting families and building community. The poem is beautifully literal in its sentiment about sharing food, but importantly metaphoric about the coming together of our families, friends and communities, who all have a voice at the table. The act of gathering is an important human function, to share teachings, values and morals, and to help one another. My favourite line in the poem references our human vulnerability and the role our families have in holding us, all while at the kitchen table.

I had to put myself back together again recently and it was at the kitchen table that it happened. Slowly over two years, my family, friends and community helped to do this, with coffee and dreams.

My grandmother's table is still there, she is ninety-six now. It still holds conversation and dreams, sometimes now between my grandmother and my grandfather, who passed away thirty-one years ago.

It's all these experiences that have drawn me to work in health and higher education and to understand how our environments, systems and contexts influence our wellness. Our attention to place and how it functions in relation to our health has been a central focus of my work over the years.

SANDRA EADES

My personal journey into health care began early in my life. As a ten-year-old, when we took it in turns answering the teacher's question about our life ambitions, I told my Mount Barker primary school class that I wanted to be a doctor when I grew up. I came from a family of carers. My mother cared for her mother. She would walk around the corner to Nan's house every evening and rub her with goanna oil or other liniment to help relieve her pain from arthritis. I watched this daily ritual with fascination. As well, many of my mother's sisters and cousins worked as nurses' aides in hospitals in Perth or Mount Barker or elsewhere in Western Australia during the 1950s and 60s.

Growing up in Mount Barker in the 1970s was both wonderful and sad. Wonderful because we lived on Country and experienced the full embrace of our wide extended family. For the first time we had rights and could live in town, after the years of living segregated from other Australians on the Mount Barker and Cranbrook

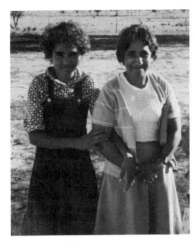

Gwen Eades with her daughter Sandra, Western Australia, ca. 1975.

native reserves. We also experienced the wonder of Country, being out in the bush whenever we had time. We were growing up in one of Australia's biodiversity hot spots and in the spring we would count endless orchids and other plants that bloomed on our land. It was sad because the pall of sickness and death was everywhere. The first time I learned of death was when I was five years old. My father was the only one of five people in a car to die after a crash just outside of Mount Barker. He left behind my pregnant mother and six children, including me. At his funeral, for the first time in my life I felt faint and overwhelmed.

My father's family helped care for us after his passing. We spent school holidays in Cranbrook with Nan Ella and Pop Sidney, where their house faced out onto Country on the outskirts of town. They had friends visit from Kalgoorlie who were Aboriginal healers in their community, and Nan never missed an opportunity to have the healers check out any of the kids or adults she thought were unwell. I suffered from childhood epilepsy that resolved as I grew older. The healers would put their hands on me and use touch to heal my liver and other parts of my body where I had illness. Pop was sick one year with the flu and wasn't expected to survive. Nan had the healers come down from Kalgoorlie to try to break the sickness. Within hours of their visit, Pop was sitting up in the hospital bed talking to the family. Throughout my life I have valued and understood the role of Aboriginal healers.

Our family continued to experience more sickness and death after my father's passing. Every year brought new sadness. Interspersed with the sadness and loss was time on Country – walking Country, talking on Country and being nurtured and healed by Country. The adults would worry on the grey misty, rainy days. They called this 'death rain' and worried that we would lose someone else. We grew up feeling our lives were intertwined with the land and weather of Country. At the passing of a relative, we all had to sit in quietness with no radio, no TV and no talking, and no naming the person we had lost. A slow train of relatives would arrive at my nan or my mum's house and, without talking, embrace the Elders and sit for hours with us. When her brother died, my mother took me to the quiet, dusty country town mortuary with her sister and some other kids to view his pale, still body. I wondered about this over the years and found that this was cultural, to have no separation or shielding of kids from the reality of death.

My nan Muriel on my mother's side of the family was soon to pass as well. She developed cancer and made many trips to Perth for treatment. Mum would travel to the city to visit her in hospital, taking all seven of her children on an overnight train ride on the *Albany Progress*. We sat on the steps of the Royal Perth Hospital for many days while the adults went in to sit with Nan. Years later, as a young doctor, I briefly worked at Royal Perth Hospital. At the time of Nan's death, we were back at home in Mount Barker. The grand matriarch was gone; she had died in the saddest way in a sterile hospital, away from home and Country and separated from her family.

Other relatives continued to die. I can't quite understand how my mother coped. She seemed to be always hopeful, always happy, and a kind and loving person. She worked as a preschool teacher's aide in the Noongar kindy (or preschool), and on occasions travelled to Perth for a week or so at a time for training related to her work. In the late 1970s, Mum decided there would be better education opportunities for the kids if we moved to Boorloo (Perth). We set off on a grand adventure that took us away from Country, from our own special part of Minang Noongar Boodja (Noongar Country), and onto the lands of Whadjuk Noongar people. The climate was different, the bush was different and the waterways and landmarks were different. We often returned home on holidays to walk on our own special Country, where the adults knew every water hole, every landmark, every good place to hunt and fish. We knew we still belonged, but we had a new home for a time.

As a high-school student attending one of Perth's poorest schools in the 1980s, I told my career counsellor I was interested in working in health care when I left school. The school called up the Perth Aboriginal Medical Service (PAMS) and asked them if they would take me as a work-experience student, and they agreed. I caught the bus into the city each day for two weeks to go to the PAMS building in East Perth. When I walked through the doors as a fifteen-year-old, it was the first time in my life that I'd entered an organisation run by Aboriginal people for Aboriginal people. My mother's cousin, Uncle Denis Hayward, was the Chief Executive Officer of the PAMS. I met the beautiful Florence Springs, an Aboriginal nurse who supervised my work experience initially, and doctors Raji Krishnan and David Paul, who worked there at the time.

Florence gave me the job of relabelling all the paper-based medical records as part of upgrading their medical records. Through this, I became familiar with the names of many Noongar people across Perth. Florence and other nurses took me with them into clinic rooms when they administered vaccinations or changed wound dressings and provided other care. I recall how relaxed and happy the patients and staff were in the organisation. Later in the week, I was moved to reception and worked answering phone calls to the clinic and checking in new patients.

Two years later, at the end of 1984, I finished high school and I was accepted to study medicine at the University of Newcastle in New South Wales. My friends at the Perth Aboriginal Medical Service were thrilled to hear my news. They invited me and my mother and other family members to the PAMS to celebrate. The service presented me with a cheque of about $500 to help with my start at university. Aunty Joan Winch congratulated me and wished me well with my studies. Aunty Joan was the first Aboriginal community health nurse in Western Australia, and she set up the first Aboriginal health-worker training program in Australia.

When I graduated from medical school in 1990, I was the first Noongar person to become qualified as a doctor in Western medicine, and my community celebrated my success with me as an outstanding role model, demonstrating Aboriginal people's ability to lead in health care. My mother took a long train trip across the country to attend my graduation.

I am sure my early contact with health leaders in my community, such as Uncle Denis Hayward and Aunty Joan Winch, helped strengthen my understanding of how Aboriginal control worked towards better health services for our mob.

When I applied for the university entry as a seventeen-year-old, I was interviewed by Professor Robert Sanson-Fisher, one of the most important professors in the Medical Faculty. He asked me why I wanted to study medicine. I told him my mother's stories about how hard it was for her mother to receive care for her invasive cancer and how my grandmother felt uncomfortable in hospital surrounded by white people who didn't fully understand her and her needs. I said I wanted to be part of the system of health care to ensure Noongar people like my grandmother had better care in the future. I was shy and had difficulty answering all the questions I was asked that day. My mother attended the interview with me, and Professor Sanson-Fisher asked her if she thought I could cope with medical school and living away from home. She replied that of course I could; I was always good at achieving what I set my mind to do. In due course

I completed the remaining on-campus aspects of the selection process and was elated to receive an offer to commence my first year of medicine in 1985. The rest, as they say, is history.

It is now almost forty years since I walked into a medical school. In the early 2000s, I graduated with a PhD in Medicine from the University of Western Australia. My mother and brother Stafford attended my graduation, sitting in the front row to watch the ceremony. Fiona Stanley and Anne Read were my supervisors. I was the first Indigenous Australian to complete a medical degree and PhD in Medicine. The things I learnt about Western medicine, combined with what I learned from my family about Country and traditional wellbeing, have filled my professional life. I loved science as a kid, and I thought of Western medicine as an applied science that was essential for ending the pain we felt as kids growing up and feeling powerless to stop the suffering that surrounded us on many days. I had a desperate desire not to lose my mother in addition to all the other remarkable adults who had shaped our lives.

My mother took us full circle to understanding the life-death-life meaning of Country and what is health. She lived a full and wonderful life. She persevered through every setback and was always hopeful, optimistic, kind and loving. She was eighty-one years old when she died. With my sisters, I took her to see her GP in Perth after she stopped eating on New Year's Day 2020. We knew she had cancer, and we knew this cancer had spread to her liver. Her GP wanted to send her to hospital for care, but she said, 'No, I want to go home.' So we brought her home and called Silverchain, the palliative care service, to help with her care.

Mum was surrounded by family at home during her last days of life. When her GP came to check on her, he said he knew which house was hers because of the many cars parked outside, making it look like a used car lot. I told everyone who came to visit Mum to make sure they came early or late and spent time alone with her. She would have something she wanted to say to each one of us. The beauty of dying at home on Country was that we were in control and the cultural aspects of care were intertwined with the need for Western medicines. I rubbed Mum's body with balm, just the way I witnessed her rub her mother's body with goanna oil from years before.

I was exhausted caring for Mum with my sisters and by the time she was close to death I needed to sleep and left others to care for her overnight. I expected someone to wake me when she passed. I woke early to the sounds of the birds as the sun was rising and thought I should get up, go see what had been happening. I walked into her bedroom where she lay, with my youngest sister and Mum's cousin sitting with her and holding vigil. From the door of the room, I could see the pulse wave from her heartbeat on the side of her neck. I called out to her good morning and walked in to sit down beside her and join the vigil. Within two minutes I could no longer see that pulse wave in her neck. I leaned down and put my head on her chest and then knew her heart had stopped beating. It was a sad but sacred moment, filled with the spirit of our ancestors throughout time.

A little later I walked out of the room full of sadness into the light outside her bedroom window. In the dawn, a sole culbardi, magpie, was standing looking around. My mother's totem, the culbardi, and our symbol of sadness was there to speak, linked to Country to mark her time to rejoin her ancestors. The ancestors always told us one magpie for sadness and two magpies for happiness. Country was true on the saddest of all days; it was life, death, and now we waited for new life.

FIONA STANLEY

I was born in Sydney and lived near La Perouse for the first ten years of my life. We came to know the Timbery family who lived at the 'native' settlement there, and Joe Timbery tried to teach my brother and me to throw the boomerang! Joe was an expert and during the 1954 Royal Tour, he threw the boomerang for the Queen. Although I knew some Aboriginal people in my early years, when we moved to a privileged white Perth suburb, in 1956, I had no contact with them. We collected clothes and other things for the Aboriginal kids who lived in the Parkerville Children's Home, but we had no idea why they were there or that they were part of the Stolen Generations. It was not until I was a medical student that I visited Aboriginal communities and began the learnings that have influenced my life and career.

At the end of my second year at university, in 1966, I had a three-month position as an unqualified nurses' aide at the Port Hedland Hospital. All future doctors should work as nurses or nurses' aides to appreciate the work they do. During that time, I went out on the weekly Flying Doctor clinics to many remote communities and towns, including Nullagine, Jigalong, Giles, Wingellina and

Wittenoom, and saw the living conditions for Aboriginal people and the diseases these conditions caused. We also had several emergencies that involved the deaths of, or serious conditions in, Aboriginal people in Port Hedland and surrounding areas in the Pilbara region. To my amazement, the then small town of Port Hedland (population 800) had a separate hospital for 'natives', which I visited on several occasions.

As a newly graduated doctor in 1970, before there were any Aboriginal medical services in Western Australia, I joined the Aboriginal Advancement Council in East Perth. I worked with a group of doctors and others in what was called the New Era Aboriginal Fellowship. This organisation resulted in the establishment of the Perth Aboriginal Medical Service (PAMS) and the WA Aboriginal Legal Service.

The overwhelming experiences for me were the two major trips in 1970 and 71 that the group of doctors organised to visit every mission, camp and town where Aboriginal people lived, from the Eastern Goldfields to the remote northwest, as far north as Kalumburu. We talked to the Elders and families about their lives and their needs, and for me it was a devastating but important learning experience. While alcohol was part of their lives, few of the women drank and it seemed to me they played a vital role in holding the families and communities together. We wrote reports with recommendations to improve living conditions.

I was also working at the Perth Children's Hospital (then called the Princess Margaret Hospital) and would try to treat the severely ill and dehydrated children who came in from these communities, often on their own without any family members with them. We would discharge them back to these environments, having performed 'medical miracles' to save them, as the local Perth newspapers would report.

This was really the beginning of my advocacy journey. I joined the Black Power movement, visited Redfern in New South Wales to see the new Aboriginal medical service there, and started to understand what racism and marginalisation meant in Western Australia and Australia more generally.

After visits to some communities in the southwest of Western Australia, where I encountered equally racist environments, I decided that I could never practise as a paediatrician. Following the preventable death of a young Aboriginal boy, I left my hospital training and fled to the UK, where I discovered social medicine, epidemiology and public health. Lights went on for me – I could continue working as a doctor, but one who was more interested in preventing diseases than treating them and seeing them come back again and again. I trained at the London School of Hygiene and Tropical Medicine, which I realised later was one of the top training centres in the world for public health.

After a final year in the USA, looking at American Indian health services as well as the top data centres for maternal, child and youth health, I returned to Western Australia in 1977 to start my research career. My whole interest was to investigate the developmental pathways to health and disease in population data in that state. It was a most exciting time as there was a scarcity of such scientific expertise in Australia; I had connections with all the best centres internationally and we managed to get funding to collect very useful data. I continued my work in Aboriginal health and worked with Ted Wilkes, the director of the Perth Aboriginal Medical Service, now called the Derbal Yerrigan, and with Dr Joan Winch, an outstanding Aboriginal nurse who set up Marr Mooditj, the first Aboriginal health-worker training centre in Australia.

After ten years establishing my research team and accruing large longitudinal data sets, I realised that to understand and improve pathways for children's wellbeing, we would need to work collaboratively. We decided to set up a multidisciplinary research institute, working with populations and communities, right through to looking at cells, genes and molecules, with the overriding focus on why children got sick and whether we could prevent problems and improve outcomes. The organisation is now called the Telethon Kids Institute.

By the late 1980s, there were several Aboriginal medical services in Western Australia. When we were planning the institute, I went to these services and said, 'We are not a service provider, but a research institute. What do you want us to be for you?' They replied, 'We want you to be our mother.' What does a mother do? She nurtures her children, gives them all the knowledge, capacity and support they need to survive in a tough world, and is always there for them. Also, she lets them lead their own lives.

Our response to this was to establish a network of Aboriginal people and groups, called Kulunga, which is the Noongar word for 'child'. Through it we would recruit and train as many Aboriginal scholars as we could. We started in 1990 and I have been on this path ever since. Over the years, I have been taught so much about

Aboriginal ways of knowing and doing. By 1995, I had come to realise that working with Aboriginal leaders, using these approaches, that is, the Aboriginal ways of knowing and doing, is the only way that outcomes in health and wellbeing will improve for Aboriginal families and communities.

Funded by a National Health and Medical Research Council (NHMRC) Capacity Building grant from 2005 to 2010, we enrolled ten outstanding Aboriginal scholars and worked with them for the first five intense years. These people then recruited a larger group of scholars and built teams around them – successfully applying for another NHMRC Centre of Research Excellence grant. They taught us about the ways of using Aboriginal Community Participation Action Research and we taught them how to successfully navigate the white (often male) dominant medical research funding pathways. It was like an explosion of capacity! The scholars became postdoctoral researchers, training more Aboriginal health professionals to work in research. They also developed international collaborations with other First Nations researchers, which was an exciting and confidence-building activity. To suddenly realise that there are similar groups of marginalised populations in many colonised countries created close bonds of understanding and learning.

These outstanding scholars have become close friends and we have worked together ever since in true and trusting partnerships. One of these scholars is Professor Sandra Eades; we are still loving working and writing together!

2

PLACE, RELATIONSHIPS AND FUTURES

SHAWANA ANDREWS

As I write these words on a cool day at the beginning of Waring – the Kulin wombat season on Wurundjeri Country – news has come from Yolŋu lands that a great leader has passed. Described by one of my own Palawa Elders as 'the most significant Aboriginal leader of our generation', Dr Yunupiŋu has left a profound legacy.[1] As leader of the Gumatj clan in Northeast Arnhem Land, Dr Yunupiŋu was known for his political activism, which began with the Yirrkala Bark Petitions and the Gove Land Rights case in the 1960s. With the aim of challenging mining companies and their access to traditional lands, Dr Yunupiŋu sought to hold governments accountable for their role in enabling mining exploitation, and later, in the 1980s, delivered the Barunga Statement. More recently, Dr Yunupiŋu was part of the Senior Advisory Group for the co-design of the Indigenous Voice to Parliament. The foundation of Dr Yunupiŋu's leadership was his Law, Country and community, and throughout his life he was a ceremonial leader and Elder.

Reflecting on a lifetime of work, the Law of the land and leadership, Dr Yunupiŋu wrote in his essay 'Rom Watangu':[2]

> What Aboriginal people ask is that the modern world now makes the sacrifices necessary to give us a real future. To relax its grip on us. To let us breathe, to let us be free of the determined control exerted on us to make us like you. And you should take that a step further and recognise us for who we are, and not who you want us to be. Let us be who we are – Aboriginal people in a modern world – and be proud of us. Acknowledge that we have survived the worst that the past had thrown at us, and we are here with our songs, our ceremonies, our land, our language and our people – our full identity. What a gift this is that we can give you, if you choose to accept us in a meaningful way.

These words describe what is meant when we refer to health: having a full identity, the authority to be who we are and to live our lives in ways that accord to our culture, Country and sustained knowledges. At his passing, Dr Yunupiŋu's family described him as '[t]he holder of our sacred fire, the leader of our clan and the path-maker to our future'.[3] In this reflection on Dr Yunupiŋu, we see three themes that speak of place, relationships and looking to new horizons.

PLACE

Place is often invisible, recognised only by those who have a relationship with it. Determined by perception, experience and relationship, place is a complex and visceral set of encounters that hold meaning through histories, languages and memories. The invisible realm that constitutes place requires reflective attentiveness for its integral role in many aspects of our lives, such as health. The invisibility of Aboriginal place to the colonial eye underlies governmental health policy and its negligible benefit for Aboriginal communities in Australia. In relation to health, place assumes a particular relevance. Aboriginal Elders, healers and health professionals remind us that Country is health. Knowledge about nutrition, medicine and healing, identity and spiritual wellbeing is traditionally sourced from Country. While some of these knowledges and the practices they inform have recently been accepted into Australia's health system, most remain invisible to it or are relegated to the periphery of 'real' medicine and health care.

Country is a distinct form of place; it is central to being Aboriginal. It transcends place; it is more than just its physical form and is described in the book *Country* as a 'continuum – without beginning or ending'.[4] Holding Law and knowledge, it is an important source of Aboriginal health and wellbeing. Country has layers of complexity and interwoven relationships with physical, ancestral and spiritual dimensions that are understood to be one. Country, in this way, is not seen as something separate from the self but rather as a living part of us, or as kin. Our identity is bound with Country and so, therefore, is our health. The wellness of people reflects the wellness of Country. Our work in caring for Country is also caring for ourselves.

If we think of the land across the continent, it is often described as red, although it comes in many colours. The ochre of the land is an expression of the way we are one with Country. Ochre is used across Australia and sits at the nexus of the earth and spiritual worlds. Red ochre is widely revered and is thought by some to represent the blood of ancestors. Wilgie Mia, or Thuwarri Thaa (the place of red ochre), is located in the Weld Ranges in Western Australia. It is a significant ochre mine that is estimated to be 27,000 years old.

It is said that:

> a [red] Kangaroo [Marlu] was wounded down near the coast. It hopped back through the country and dropped spots of blood along the way. It dropped quite a bit at Little Wilgie Mia, then it died at Wilgie Mia which left a lot of ochre. Then the spirit of the Kangaroo moved from Wilgie Mia to the hill right next-door to it.[5]

Yellow, brown, white and other shades also feature in ochre's spectrum of use as a pigment, modified from iron-rich rock through grinding, scraping and knapping.[6] Mixed with a fluid such as water, saliva, blood, or animal fat or oil, it can be applied to rock, weapons, ceremonial objects, skin and hair. Ochre is used for both ceremonial and functional reasons. The latter includes health and hygiene, for the care of wounds such as burns, for the treatment of sores and insect bites, and it is used for protection from the elements.[7] It may also be mixed with other medicinal substances such as sap, leaves, ashes or oil and then applied. Ochre's rich iron compounds and mineral content are said to have antiseptic, antacid and styptic (binding) properties.[8] White ochre is known as kaolin and was used to treat diarrhoea; it forms the basis of the medication we buy today for the same treatment.

My ancestor Mannalargenna would wear his locked hair and beard adorned with grease and ochre. He would also paint it on his skin as a symbol of his leadership among the clanspeople and his role as a cleverman and as a symbol of his Country. I don't live on Country, but on the first Saturday of December each year, my daughters and I attend Mannalargenna Day on Trouwerner (Tasmania) in the northeast, Tebrakunna Country. It is a day to honour our ancestor and to celebrate the life journey of a clan leader, warrior and powerful spirit man who played a pivotal role in the lives of the clanspeople of the Coastal Plains Nation. Mannalargenna died on 4 December 1835 at Wybalenna on Flinders Island. The day is held annually around this anniversary, and we gather to celebrate our continuing cultural connections. It is also an important day for eating foods that have sustained the Coastal Plains Nation for thousands of years, such as muttonbird, Cape Barren goose, crayfish and other seafoods, and wallaby. An important unbroken connection for those who do live on Country has been the harvesting for thousands of years of yolla, the muttonbird or short-tailed shearwater, which is valued for its meat, oil, eggs and feathers.

Aboriginal peoples across Tasmania centred their hunting strategies on both seasonal and staple resources sourced from land and sea. Much of the seafood and birdlife, including muttonbird, Cape Barren goose and seal, have a high oil content and are rich in omega-3 fatty acids, which support a healthy metabolism and heart. Balanced with other foods such as wallaby, kangaroo, possum, plant-based foods and eel, the diet provides the essential protein, fatty acids and micronutrients needed for healthy human growth and function. It also supports the physical and mental-health requirements for ongoing survival in a cold climate. Conversely, the tasks of hunting, fishing and gathering require good physical and mental health. Both place and relationships are central to these tasks to ensure the success of food production and to enable the generational learning that sustains these practices.

RELATIONSHIPS

Prior to colonisation, health was not something to be sought and attained. Health was innate through the process of living and, along with diet, was intimately connected to Country. Built on sophisticated knowledge of environments, seasons, sustainable harvesting practices, processing techniques and nutritional values, food security and nutrition don't exist in isolation but sit within a complex structure of relations. Food production is linked to the sustainability of Country and is supported through kinship and sacramental totemic systems. Totems are usually accounted for across moieties, the first order of social organisation – groups are separated into two, mirroring one another by axes of gender, generation or other social aspects, in order to distribute authority and resources evenly.[9] The responsibility to protect and care for one's totem, which includes animals, plants and natural resources, links humans with the spiritual world in an obligatory symbiotic relationship that provides and protects.

The production of food according to roles associated with gender is sometimes incorrectly assumed to be separated by a delineation between hunting and gathering. Clanswomen of Trouwerner's Coastal Plains Nation, for example, were hunters of the sea. Sea Country is women's Country, and Pairrebeenne/Trawlwoolway Elder Aunty Patsy Cameron speaks of the agility and strength of women in relation to their gathering of sea resources and economic contribution.

> In the Coastal Plains society, the role and status of females was distinct from that of males. This was evident in the skills required for a range of economic tasks. The clanswomen were the main economic providers for their families, and they claimed many gathering and collecting tasks as their own … [the] women were renowned for their strength and skills as superior swimmers and divers. Braving the cold, often turbulent and shark-infested waters, they remained submerged for long periods of time to harvest the marine resources so important to the clan's daily dietary requirements. They could swim considerable distances to

the closer offshore islands and rocky outcrops to harvest oil-rich seal and muttonbirds and collect the fine quality, tool-making stone. Along the coastal margins numerous varieties of shellfish, sea mammals and sea birds were gathered as favoured foods to complement the foodstuffs harvested on land.[10]

Leadership and authority in medicinal knowledge and healing practice are held in different ways. The basics, colloquially called 'bush medicine' today, can generally be known by everyone and are taught to children at a young age. More specialised knowledge and treatment using the pharmacological and therapeutic application of plants and botanicals might be held by Elders or people with particular healing or wellbeing roles.[11, 12] Traditional healers, clevermen, sacred knowledge keepers, seers and others with healing or medicinal skills all have exceptional knowledge and powers for healing. They heal through stories and ancestral knowledge and are often the cultural keepers of spiritual beliefs. The Ngangkari of the Ngaanyatjarra, Pitjantjatjara and Yankunytjatjara (NPY) Lands are an example of such healers. They inherit healing powers through beliefs, bloodlines and traditional training methods. The focus of Ngangkari healing practice is a person's spirit, providing care through diagnoses and treatment using techniques such as counselling and general support, massage, smoking, song and breathwork. The Ngangkari describe themselves as having 'healing hands', hands that hold mapanpa, sacred tools, and that work with the spirit.[13]

Ngangkari can work with many health problems. Mental health, or a sick spirit, is an important area they help with. Bringing their knowledge of the spiritual world and working in the context of family and community, healers of the NPY Lands play an important role in holding people and keeping them connected. This is done in the context of intimate knowledge about kinship and the place people have within it.

In *Traditional Healers of Central Australia: Ngangkari*,[14] the second publication of the Ngaanyatjarra, Pitjantjatjara and Yankunytjatjara Women's Council Aboriginal Corporation about the Ngangkari, Anangu knowledge of their traditional ways of understanding health, healing and continuity is shared. The Ngangkari who tell their stories in it speak of their powers for healing and treating all who ask. Some Ngangkari get their healing powers at a very young age and have experienced a lifetime of learning and applying their techniques. Using these techniques, such as the healing breath or singing sacred songs of healing and massage, the Ngangkari can help people become well again.

———

The knowledge Aboriginal healers hold has been cultivated since the beginning of time. Western health systems are comparatively new and are largely built on biomedical constructions of health, which are based on the presence or absence of disease, and on reductionist science.[15] The intersection of Aboriginal and Western health beliefs and systems is a complex one. In my time spent working in a large metropolitan hospital, there were numerous occasions in which the disjuncture was obvious. On one occasion, an Aboriginal mother had travelled from interstate with her child who needed urgent specialised surgery. She was distressed and would not leave her child unless an Aboriginal staff member sat with the child. The mother was anxious about the severity of the illness and because she and her child had no family there at the hospital. In the intensive care unit, the child was struggling two days after the surgery and her mum came to me to request a flight home and some time alone with her child. We talked and on the third morning, from the curtained bed, came her singing. Afterwards the child's mum advised the nursing staff that she would be leaving to go home. There was quiet outrage among the staff.

The mother had told us that her child's spirit had already left. Late on the third day, the mother left the hospital, and the state, to go home. We Aboriginal staff spent as much time sitting with the child as we could. On the fourth day, the child passed away, and arrangements were made for an interstate transfer. In her own way, the mother had upheld her spiritual beliefs in the context of a Western health system. She had shown stoic leadership in the face of grief as she guided me and the other Aboriginal staff who worked to advocate for her needs and choices. Throughout this experience, I had felt inadequate and lacking in the right knowledge. The mother had guided me through what she was experiencing, and I hope my intent to offer her some comfort and advocate for her was enough.

On another occasion, a young child was waiting for an organ transplant. Months had passed and she became more unwell, finally reaching an urgent state that meant she was moved to the top of the national transplant waiting list. The child was admitted to the intensive care unit for a number of weeks. The family situation was complex. They lived interstate, her dad could not travel and her mum had the care of other children. The child mentioned that she'd had a visit from her dad. She said that her dad visited her in the night but that it was not a dream. He spent time with her every night until she successfully received a transplant. The family confirmed that they were offering their healing from their lands.

These stories reflect the careful consideration of Aboriginal people in their engagement with two systems of health, the difficult decisions made, the negotiation of obligation and relationships and the understanding one system needs to have of the other. They also highlight the particular relationship with the spiritual world that is part of many Aboriginal people's concept of health.

FUTURES

In the western parts of Victoria, on Gunditjmara Country, the brolga dances with rhythmic grace in the cool months of late spring when the frogs sing their chorus and the orchids are flowering. Parading its elongated body across the wetlands with carefully placed footsteps, the brolga leaps into the air, wings folded and head bowing down, then up again in an exhibition of dalliance with their life partner. It is a show of confidence and optimism, demonstrating the brolgas' determination to dance themselves into the future. The show is anticipated in western Victoria as it is in other parts of the country, such as in the East Kimberley on Gija Country, where the brolga is an Ancestral Being who connects people with Country and ancestors through time, bringing into being all that is connected to Gija landscape.[16]

Futures are stories that have not yet taken place. They are full of possibilities. Future stories can free us from the narratives that oppress and marginalise us. They can transgress the confines of time and history and can survive even if not told or realised. Our futures are forged according to our histories. The challenge for the leaders of our time – the path-makers – and our health is how we understand and act upon where we have come from and where we are going. Seeing our path-makers' visions reflected in health policy and across all levels of the health system is important to connecting two sets of health understandings.

In 1989, a landmark document in Aboriginal and Torres Strait Islander health policy was produced by the National Aboriginal Health Strategy Working Group. For the first time, a national approach to Aboriginal and Torres Strait Islander health was considered and the 1989 National Aboriginal Health Strategy (NAHS) was developed from an extensive consultative process that identified Aboriginal and Torres Strait Islander peoples' health aspirations and principles for achieving these within a rights-based policy framework.[17] The strategy described health as:

> a matter of determining all aspects of their [Aboriginal people's] life, including control over their physical environment, of dignity, of community self-esteem and of justice. It is not merely a matter of the provision of doctors, hospitals, medicines or the absence of disease and incapacity.

This was later developed into a working definition of health that is still used today:

> Not just the physical well-being of the individual but the social, emotional, and cultural well-being of the whole community. This is a whole-of-life view and it also includes the cyclical concept of life-death-life.

At that time, there were a number of Aboriginal community-controlled health organisations that had already been set up to deliver primary health care to their local communities. The Aboriginal Medical Service in Redfern, the Victorian Aboriginal Health Service and Central Australian Aboriginal Congress, for example, were established in the 1970s, to address significant unmet health needs in Aboriginal communities. The wreckage caused by colonisation created significant damage to community wellness. Loss of relationships between people, land and traditional belief systems created a collective loss that communities themselves worked hard to meet in a climate of discrimination and marginalisation. If you have ever been in an Aboriginal health service you will understand how these are not just service providers, they are places of gathering where community can be together. Being able to gather, particularly during times of trauma or displacement, is important; it nurtures the spirit and strengthens relationships. This is what underpins the Aboriginal community-controlled health sector and it's what you see and feel in these organisations. The National Aboriginal Health

Strategy, in its preamble, linked colonisation to poor Aboriginal health and the community-controlled health sector was responding to this and reaching into the future.

Casting sight towards our horizons is something that Indigenous peoples do worldwide, determining that today's decisions are accountable to the generations of the future and understanding the genealogy of all things.

In 2018, the late Dr Moana Jackson delivered the Dungala Kaiela Oration at the Rumbalara Football and Netball Club, an annual event held on Yorta Yorta Country in Shepparton, Victoria. His lecture, 'At home on Country, at home in the world', explored the United Nations' drafting of the Rights of Indigenous Peoples, and its desire to allow Indigenous people to determine their own destinies. A key message in the oration was the importance of adaptation, noting that this does not mean submission, but rather the opposite, continuing a tradition of a dynamic culture that shifts and weaves to respond to the world around us. It means directing Aboriginal attention to planning for a future that is strong enough to preserve our self-determination, flexible enough to offer those who came later a place on our lands and visionary enough to imagine a different future.[18]

As the brolgas dance for their future, so too are Aboriginal peoples all over the country working to adapt to this new world. They are building ancient knowledge systems into contemporary constructs such as community-controlled organisations and negotiating the constraints of the Western world to bridge understandings of health and to place people at the forefront of this work. Path-makers and way finders have a tough gig, charged with the task of taking carriage of our futures, their patience a virtue, as the future is not pressured to being pulled into the present.

3

BIRTHING ON COUNTRY AND DYING ON COUNTRY

FIONA STANLEY

The power of giving birth on Country relates to Mother Earth knowing that a child of a certain totem has been born and will be protected and nurtured by 'her'. Similarly, the desire of Aboriginal and Torres Strait Islander people to return to Country to die is strong, and increasingly those in the final stages of their lives request this. I have talked with many Elders who are sick and their medical requirements mean they have to live in major centres many kilometres from their Country. One of them, Aunty Tootsie Daniels, is a matriarch of the Yindjibarndi people from Roebourne. This is Murujuga Country, where Tootsie and others are fighting to save

Australia's largest collection of petroglyphs, on the Burrup Peninsula where the Woodside gas hub is situated. To have dialysis for her renal failure, she has to stay in Perth or Port Hedland three days a week.

Tootsie is lobbying for more dialysis machines to be available on Country, so that she and others in the same situation do not have to be away from the land and the people they love.[1] This is a deeply spiritual connection – Aboriginal identity is intimately bound to Country, and ceremonies on Country while birthing or dying and in the time after death are considered crucial.

This resurgent interest in bringing back traditional practices at both the beginning and end of life in Aboriginal communities across Australia is reflected in movements that are taking place worldwide.[2]

GATHERING THE SEEDS SYMPOSIUM AND BIRTHING SERVICES

My interests and experience lie mostly in the early years of life, so my knowledge of birthing and child health is more complete than my understandings of dying on Country. I was privileged to attend the *Gathering the Seeds* Symposium, held in Perth in April 2023, which provided a very broad and deep overview of Birthing on Country philosophies and programs in Australia. As well, by talking with Noongar Elders Millie and Fred Penny, I have now learned more about dying on Country. Western thinking tends to compartmentalise these aspects of life, but Aboriginal people do not view them as separate events; dying is part of the circle of life, which starts at conception. So let us start in early life too.

The *Gathering the Seeds* birthing symposium was organised by three outstanding Indigenous professors – Rhonda Marriott from Murdoch University and Cath Chamberlain and Marcia Langton, both from Melbourne University.[3] The national *Replanting the Birthing Trees* Commonwealth-funded research project was launched at the symposium.[4] Over three days, Indigenous maternal and child health professionals gave presentations describing how they are combining traditional Grandmothers' Way of Birthing with Western medicine to provide a trusted, culturally nurturing service for Indigenous women giving birth today, such as the Koori Maternity Service,[5] Boodjari Yorgas,[6] and Birthing on Noongar Boodjar.[7]

The official artwork for the symposium, *Replanting the Birth Trees*, painted in 2022 by Valerie Ah Chee, appeared on all our bags, t-shirts and cards. (You can see the painting on the inside front cover of this book.) Valerie Ah Chee is also a midwife, and provided an explanation of the artwork:

> This artwork represents the strength and resilience of Aboriginal and Torres Strait Islander people in respect to our birthing and parenting over the generations. The tree is strong and healthy and has strong roots that are embedded deeply in Country, culture and family. The trunk is strong, sturdy and enduring and a family is represented here: pregnant mother, father and child supported by the roots and each person, an integral part of community. In the top left corner, we start with communities, represented by circles that make up the foliage of the tree. This foliage starts out grey and muted with pops of colour representing our traditional

knowledge, birth rites and practices emerging from trauma and hardship, knowledge that has always been there, but has been lying dormant until the time was right to emerge. As this foliage moves across to the right, it blooms with strength, health and colour and is connected to form a beautiful and vibrant canopy, supported by the sturdy trunk and ancient roots. This foliage drops seeds so that other trees, the saplings seen here, can grow and stand strong. The grey circles on the black background represent the birthing places all over this land, connecting us again to Country. In the earth, the circles represent the continuing birthing women, from generation to generation, unbroken with the smaller circles above and below representing our knowledge and strength as energy, passed on from our grandmothers and is never ending. At the bottom of the picture are our ancestors, men and women, born from Country and passing back into Country, holding us up, protecting us and making us strong. In our lives we tap into this strength from our ancestors to keep us moving forward.[8]

The birthing services discussed at the symposium all have similar philosophies and ways of working. All were established by Aboriginal women and their families, with important input from the female Elders who hold the knowledge of Grandmothers' Laws and Ways of birthing. They employ highly trained Aboriginal staff in all areas – midwives, health workers, administrative staff – with Elders and other family members, to ensure a culturally safe environment. Most incorporate dedicated non-Indigenous midwives and other staff to ensure that, given their risk factors, the Aboriginal women have the best of both services. As Galiwin'ku Elder Rosemary Gundjarraŋbuy said at the symposium, 'We are sharing knowledge – walking hand in hand.'

The objective of these services is to improve outcomes by providing a range of vital support progams, which start from before pregnancy. These services include sexual and reproductive, family planning, antenatal and childbirth education, breastfeeding and postnatal care and parenting support. The aims are to help Aboriginal women to birth in hospitals, embedding culture and health promotion with continuity across all aspects of pregnancy care; help high-risk families; broker good relationships with health-care professionals, specialists and others; and build trust. Some, such as the Koori Maternity Services[9] and SWAMS Boodjari Moort/Kwilenap,[10] exist within Aboriginal community-controlled health services. They are holistic and family centred and offer a range of other services such as dental care, nutrition, stopping smoking, housing support, recovery from substance abuse, domestic violence support services, and transport to appointments. Even those that are 'stand-alone', such as Boodjari Yorgas,[11] broker partnerships with important mainstream or other Aboriginal services to provide all the help that families with new babies need for their children to receive the best support.

Partnerships and collaborations are at the centre of these services: between the Aboriginal birthing services and all other services, and between the families and the staff. These models have also influenced how mainstream services offer care to their Aboriginal clients and even to those non-Aboriginal women who want the nurturing and continuity of care.

The theme of relationships – caring, respectful, trusting and understanding – is common throughout this book about how Aboriginal people can participate in the mainstream culture and take the best of both worlds.

The first such birthing service was Congress Alukura in Alice Springs. It was established in 1986 from the Aboriginal Medical Service Congress, to implement Grandmothers' Way of Birthing for women in that region.[12] I recall being in Alice Springs to support Congress and the mothers in this new venture, but the white obstetrician at the hospital was not happy (in spite of being a woman!). It took some time for other traditional birthing services to be developed across the country. The Birthing on Country movement in Australia is now increasing in strength and capacity, as more and more Aboriginal women are lobbying for it and more Aboriginal women are trained in those areas relevant to supporting birthing. There is also an enlightened group of non-Indigenous midwives, researchers and other professionals who are strong allies of this movement.

Professors Yvette Roe and Sue Kildea have been leaders in designing and evaluating Birthing on Country for some years. They jointly direct the Molly Wardaguga Research Centre, which is named after a beloved Burarra Elder and Aboriginal midwife from Maningrida in the Northern Territory, who contributed significantly to the Birthing on Country movement. The centre is at Charles Darwin University, with excellent networks across the north of Australia, in both urban and rural settings. Their collaboration has been a major factor in the success of the Birthing on Country movement.

Yvette is a Jawuru woman from Western Australia, with a PhD and training in public health, midwifery and sociology. Sue Kildea is a highly regarded non-Indigenous midwifery researcher, not only researching Birthing on Country with Yvette, but willing to share leadership roles and capacity with Indigenous staff. This collaboration between Aboriginal birthing leaders and non-Aboriginal allies has occurred across Australia and has been instrumental in increasing the acceptance of Birthing on Country by governments, funders and universities. Roe and Kildea's work includes establishing and evaluating Birthing on Country in the remote Northern Territory[13] and in urban settings as well.[14]

The strength of the centre's work derives from best-practice co-design and rigorous evaluation with many published papers. These studies showed that *modern* Grandmothers' Way of Birthing programs increased attendance at antenatal care, reduced preterm birth from 14.3 per cent to 8.9 per cent, increased breastfeeding and had fewer babies admitted to intensive care.[15]

Comments from some of the women from the Koori Maternity Services suggest that the women were clearly supportive of the midwives being available throughout the pregnancy and birth. For example, 'The midwives were there all the time and they listened to you.'

'She makes you feel welcome you know, like she's not a midwife or medical staff, she makes you feel like she's family, like it was someone I've known for many years – like I could open up to her and tell her what was going on in my life.'

'I think the program's great where women have got the midwives to connect with. Having that connection with the workers is important. I think it's really beautiful and you just get to trust that person. It makes mums feel special.'

'I don't know how to explain it, it was like they gave you more time, they actually cared about you and the baby, they didn't make it out like you were just another patient like they can just shove you on your way ... and I have had that before.'[16]

Sue Kildea and Yvette Roe summarised the essentials of these services as RISE – **Redesign** the service; **Invest** in the workforce (Aboriginal); **Strengthen** families; and **Embed** in Aboriginal and Torres Strait Islander governance and control.[17] An excellent article summarising the positive impacts of Australian Aboriginal traditional birthing was presented in the prestigious medical journal *The Lancet*.[18] The exciting observation is that because Aboriginal pregnant women and mothers trust the service, they use it. Attendance rates for antenatal care and for preventive services have increased dramatically compared with those for Aboriginal women in mainstream services. There is now clear evidence that Birthing on Country services reduce, by 60 per cent, the risk of children being taken into care,[19,20] affirming the power of culture to enhance the confidence and capacity of families.

Birthing on Country or traditional birthing relates to how the service is set up, not that women are necessarily going back on Country to have their babies. While they are not on their ancestral lands – in fact, many give birth away from Country – the service reflects those aspects of Grandmothers' Way of Birthing that make it so accepted and nurturing.

> Birthing on Country is a metaphor for the best start in life for Aboriginal and Torres Strait Islander babies and their families and is an integrated, holistic and culturally appropriate model of care for all. Key elements include but are not limited to: i) Aboriginal governance; ii) continuity of midwifery care during pregnancy, birth and beyond; iii) direct access to specialised women's health, paediatric and social and emotional wellbeing services; iv) intensive support for vulnerable women and families; (v) improved integration between mainstream and community-controlled health sector.[21]

Aboriginal and Torres Strait Islander women have poor perinatal outcomes compared with non-Indigenous women, with higher rates of both maternal and child mortality and of preterm and low birthweight births. And we know that birthweight influences health over the course of one's life. High rates of diseases resulting from historical government policies and current living conditions, such as diabetes, heart disease, mental-health problems, substance abuse, anaemia and infections, are harmful for Aboriginal mums and their babies.

Distrust in mainstream services and institutional racism have powerful negative impacts on pregnant women and their families. Aboriginal women have spoken of their birth experiences in mainstream hospitals and facilities. They tell of racial stereotyping, of women being sent from the hospital building to give birth in old sheds, on verandahs, and often in fear and with serious neglect. With few exceptions, their stories were very different from the experiences of how their own mothers had given birth in the warmth and nurturing of the traditional and trusted 'old ways'.

For some families who live remotely, the Western medical services insist that pregnant women, many of whom are young, scared and poorly prepared, travel to major centres many weeks before their due date, to deliver 'safely'. In reality, this clinical decision means they do not have the social support of their family or community. Also, facing stigma from mainstream professionals, they do not feel safe and their spiritual and emotional wellbeing suffers. Many women will try to avoid using these services again. Stories from those who have given birth in urban mainstream services tell of the hostile ways in which the women are managed and made to feel unworthy and inferior. If they try to ask for some changes in treatment, their medical notes may report 'Uncooperative Aboriginal patient'. There is often also an ignorance on the doctors' part that is disrespectful, as this quote from an Aboriginal woman in Melbourne who was pregnant for the first time shows: 'The doctor asked me if "ATSI" [Aboriginal and Torres Strait Islander] was a disease. He had no idea what it meant. He was trying hard to be respectful but was ignorant. He continued to ask questions and his preconceived ideas were bizarre. I didn't enjoy the scan, I felt uncomfortable and had to give a history lesson and explain myself.'[22]

Not only do new Birthing on Country services have to disassociate their services from European ways of birthing, they also must counter the dependence on largely white male obstetricians and the juggernaut of invasive obstetrics that has occurred in mainstream services. Male obstetricians and hospitals have radically changed birthing in all developed and increasingly developing countries from births at home managed by groups of experienced women, midwives and doulas. The changes have resulted in pregnancy and birth being considered as illnesses that demand medical intervention throughout pregnancy and delivery. Some of these interventions have been unnecessary and some harmful, and overall, they have taken away the social and nurturing aspects of women's pregnancy, labour and delivery. Modern obstetrics is focused exclusively on the baby's survival. Aboriginal birthing is attempting to bring back nurturing approaches to ensure that women feel that they are listened to and are part of the process.

As well, technology is being used to engage with Aboriginal families. Two examples are the digital platform *Baby Coming You Ready?*,[23] and the website SMS4Dads,[24] which is specifically for Aboriginal fathers. Once a dad or soon-to-be dad has joined the program, he is sent regular texts that are synchronised to the stage of pregnancy or development of the child. The program commences at twelve weeks gestation and continues through to the first twelve months of the baby's life. It encourages men to walk alongside their partner and support her through pregnancy and after the birth.

Increasing numbers of non-Indigenous women are unhappy with the current Australian mainstream birthing services. As they hear about these wrap-around and caring services, they wonder whether *all* services should be like these!

This is a beautiful story about a placenta garden that was established by women from the Wathaurong Nation (Geelong) in Victoria. Traditional knowledge of burying placentas had been lost by the Wathaurong women, but they were told how to do this by Yolŋu women from Gove in the Northern Territory, whose knowledge was still strong. The two groups came together when the Koori women attended a birthing conference in Arnhem Land. Even if the baby was not born on Country, the Yolŋu women explained, burying the placenta enabled the baby to grow up strong.

Back in Geelong, the Koori women asked the hospital staff to freeze their placentas until the garden was established. This story demonstrates how Aboriginal people adapt old ways to a Western setting.[25]

The Wathaurong Women's Tranquillity Garden was created on Wathaurong land and kept safe and secure with a brush wall and locked gate. The local Bunnings store sent their female staff to help landscape and plant the garden. The first ceremony to plant the placentas that had been stored was in 2011; all the mums, children, nanas, aunties and friends were invited to come along. Forty placentas were buried that day, and the garden has been flourishing ever since. Each burial ceremony starts with a story about how the garden came about, and next to the Birth Tree are the words:

> This is our birth tree, like our lives it is always changing. In autumn the leaves change colour, in spring the leaves grow back and in summer the tree flowers. Sometimes in our lives we have difficult times and it can be tough to work through. But like our

birth tree each phase is needed to be able to go on to the next. In winter the tree looks the worse for wear but without it we wouldn't have the beautiful summer flowers. Our lives are a journey and our experiences make us who we are today. The placenta we are planting today has nourished and grown this beautiful bubba and now it will nourish our birth tree.

We would like to welcome baby to the Wathaurong Community. Our hopes and dreams for baby are to grow up healthy and strong and well connected to Country and Culture.

They have now planted over 100 placentas and the garden has become a special place for women. It is peaceful, and women and their children can go there to get respite and feel safe. As well, the staff sometimes use it for counselling. It is particularly therapeutic for grieving mothers who have lost a baby or whose child is subsequently removed. They can feel the connection to Country, which provides some comfort and healing. Dr Jill Gallagher, the CEO of the Victorian Aboriginal Community Controlled Health Organisation (VACCHO), says:

The placenta is a beautiful organ. It is responsible for growing a healthy baby. It is the bridge between a mother and her baby in the womb, it is unique, amazing and beautiful. By burying the placenta it's like giving back to Mother Earth to let her know that a child has been born, so that Mother Earth can continue to nurture that Boorai [child], in particular the spiritual soul of that little person. When I had my two Boorais I was not given the option of having my placentas nor did I have a garden to bury them [in], and this makes me feel very sad. I believe all women should have that offered to them.[26]

The Ngangk Waangening (Birthing on Noongar Boodja) Project was run out of Ngangk Yira Institute for Change in Western Australia. It was conducted over a five-year period to identify from Noongar Elders the service gaps, issues and barriers for Aboriginal women in the mainstream maternity care services. It was driven by the same needs as the other examples in this chapter: Aboriginal women feeling unwelcome and undermined by the mainstream services, with staff having little understanding of their lived experiences and the impact of history on their lives. I am honoured to be the Patron of Ngangk Yira and on the advisory panel for this project.

The report *Birthing on Noongar Boodjar-Ngangk Waangening*[27] is being used to inform a co-designed maternity service – their recommendations are based on the following principles:

1. Aboriginal women across the whole of Western Australia should have equitable access to culturally secure service providers with a culturally competent health service.
2. That care be centred on mothers and their families.
3. There be a commitment to employ Aboriginal people in all areas – practice, diagnosis, support and administration.
4. Indigenous data sovereignty [*see* chapter 9] be used to evaluate – obtaining the best data to measure, longitudinally, how well the mothers and babies are doing.

The Boodjari Moort/Kwilenap (Noongar name for 'place of the dolphins') is the maternal and child health clinic run out of the South West Aboriginal Medical Service (SWAMS) in Bunbury, southwest of Western Australia. This holistic service provides support from the start of pregnancy to six weeks postpartum, employing midwives and Indigenous health workers, with a focus on a positive birth experience. It also offers support for domestic violence, substance abuse and playgroups for families. Lesley Nelson, CEO of SWAMS, said at the *Gathering the Seeds* Symposium: 'Every Aboriginal child deserves a champion – an adult or an organisation that will never give up on them, who understands the power of connection, family, community and culture, and helps them become the best version of themselves within a culturally appropriate and safe environment.'[28]

The Birthing on Country programs summarised above are successful because they have been developed, designed and implemented by Aboriginal women. And because the Aboriginal health professionals are fully trained in both worlds, they bring the best of medical care to the services. They marry a trusted way of caring for women during pregnancy, delivery and after the birth with the diagnostic and therapeutic skills needed to treat diseases that were unknown in precolonial times. At present, these bold and innovative programs are significantly underfunded and unappreciated by the mainstream culture's health services and governments.

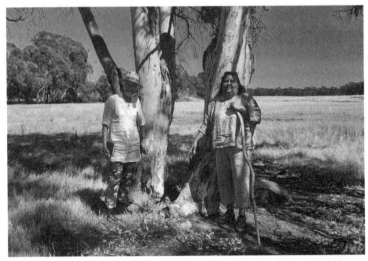

Professor Marion Kickett, a Ballardong woman from York, Western Australia, with Fiona Stanley in front of one of the birthing trees in York, November 2023. The last traditional birth there was in the 1840s.

DYING ON COUNTRY

Noongar Elders Millie (nee Walley) and Fred Penny have taught me so much about dying on Country. Millie is from Pinjarra Country, and still has strong links to her land.

On 28 October 1834, Captain James Stirling and twenty-five men ambushed a group of eighty Noongar men, women and children, today known as the Pinjarra massacre. Pinjarra's cemetery is opposite the massacre site, where a plaque has been erected. Millie's five-year-old sister Pam died in Pinjarra from a respiratory illness, and Millie and her sisters Kay and Marie and their families, who all now live in the southern suburbs of Perth, visit her grave in the cemetery every year on the day of her death and talk together about her. The three sisters have been doing this for nearly sixty years. This illustrates the importance to Millie of being able to visit where her sister Pam is buried. The Pennys and I talked about the significance of burial and ceremony around Aboriginal deaths.

Fred explained that while all people want to die on Country, those closer to their own Country and who have not moved into cities have a more 'strict culture' (more traditional) and could not contemplate not dying on Country. Depending on where your Country is and how close or far you are from services, however, culture sometimes must adapt if people need to have palliative care, renal dialysis or other Western medicine. There are challenges in providing end-of-life care to sick Aboriginal people on Country, far from cities and services – and these are not just practical and financial challenges. Very often, Western medical and nursing staff do not appreciate the practices and beliefs that are important at this time in a person's life. In some communities, for example, the preferred care is given by matrilineal relatives, so any palliative care services need to acknowledge this.[29]

Fred spoke of the many reasons why urban Aboriginal people might no longer be able to go back to die on Country or even be buried on Country – either the Country of their birth or of their ancestors. One was financial. Many families cannot afford to have services on Country, nor can they afford a funeral there. Another reason is that many want to be buried close to family, so their family can visit them; or their families want them to be buried close to where most of the family live. And if the family moved to the city, there may be two generations there. The power of family and remaining close to family after death is important and may override the dream of going back to Country to die or be buried.

Millie's paternal family come from Meekatharra, a small town 750 kilometres northeast of Perth. Her older sister was very sick in Perth and when she was dying she urged her family and caregivers to bring her back to Meekatharra to die and be buried on Country. 'She could not imagine dying anywhere else,' Millie said. The family took her to Geraldton Hospital – a big centre on the coast, with full medical facilities. And days before she died, they were able to bring her to the small hospital in Meekatharra. Her sister's family left the hospital soon after she died, just as the sun was rising, and they recall it as being very beautiful and peaceful.

Another relative who was also part of the Walley family from Meekatharra, was described by Millie as a 'bush woman'. She was diagnosed with cancer but refused treatment, remaining in the Meekatharra hospital, where she died on Country with family around her. This decision was counter to advice from Western services, which would have meant that she would have died in an urban hospital away from kin and Country.

Noongar people imagine life and death as a circle and not linear as many non-Indigenous people do. Fred Penny drew a diagram with a series of concentric circles getting smaller and smaller. If you were more distantly related to the person who had died, you would be in the outside circle, but if you were a close relative, you were in the middle of the concentric circles. He then drew a straight arrow to demonstrate our Western linear thinking, which cuts across all the circles, ignoring who is in each one.

Millie mentioned that if a relative could not get back to Pinjarra (or Meekatharra) to die or be buried, the family would bring a bucket of Pinjarra (or Meekatharra) soil for the burial in the metropolitan area. Thus, the journey to death connects strongly to Country and Mother Earth. 'We feel part of Country and Mother Earth and these knowledges have been passed on from our ancestors,' Millie said.

The beliefs and activities around Aboriginal people dying vary considerably, reflecting differences in the cultures of Indigenous peoples (which differ across the language groups in Australia), and the varying cultural adaptations made since contact and settlement, including the influence of Christianity and missions. As Fred described above and others have noted,[30] the longer people have lived away from Country, the more likely they are to modify their practices. Those closest in both time and place to ancestral lands, such as those in remote communities, are more likely to follow their traditional practices. As with knowledge about birthing, it is remarkable that in spite of the genocidal history, so many communities have retained the knowledge to follow and participate in these activities. There is a universal belief that you are born from Country, Dreaming and Songlines, and your spirit returns there. This means that where you die and where you are buried are of great importance.

It is crucial for Aboriginal people to know when the death of a family member is imminent, so they can care appropriately for the person and prepare for their death and its aftermath. In Arnhem Land and the Central Desert, where traditional practices are largely still observed, the dead person's spirit is encouraged to depart permanently from this world.[31] Various ritual processes are carried out to ensure that the spirit does not come back. This is a powerful reason for the repatriation of human remains from museums around the world, where bodies have been taken without permission over the last 200 years.

A common ritual is the naming taboo; the name of the deceased is not spoken or written by anyone for a prescribed period following the person's death. Permission to publish images or names must be sought from the Elders. Smoking and cleansing ceremonies are still important, to weaken the ties of the dead with the land of the living. In Central Australia, these activities are performed by the Ngangkari, who have special powers of healing, who combine the Western roles of physician, therapist, priest, coroner and judge.[32]

As described above, the places where people are conceived, born, live and die are of great spiritual importance to them. Most have an Ancestral Being or totem allotted to them at conception or birth and their spirit is derived from the spiritual essence of this Ancestral Being. Death is conceived as the reverse process, a stage of life rather than an event defined in time and place: 'a gentle leaching of the body and spirit back into the earth'.[33]

The provision of end-of-life care varies enormously depending on these variations in current beliefs and practices. For many urbanised Aboriginal people, access to palliative care, renal dialysis and other end-of-life interventions are relatively easy to obtain and can be incorporated around the spiritual needs of the families. In remote communities, where traditional culture is strong and following it is vital, the provision of any Western medicine is very challenging. Families with sick relatives in remote communities usually have to move off Country and away from land and families at a time when they are needed more than ever. There needs to be careful planning of services, such as dialysis, so that those wanting to die remotely can do so without excessive pain or discomfort.

Purple House is an innovative Indigenous-owned and run health service operating from its Alice Springs base. It has eighteen remote clinics and a mobile dialysis unit called the Purple Truck, and provides social support, aged-care and NDIS services. Purple House aims to get people with chronic disease back home so that families and culture can remain strong.[34]

One former director of Purple House says:

> Central Australia has gone from having the worst to the best survival rates for dialysis in Australia. We are getting more patients back home so that families and culture can remain strong. Anangu like the open space on their land, where they can smell the Spirit, the wildflowers and other plants. They want fire for the smell of wood smoke going through the air. They want to smell the flowers after rain.[35]

The Purple House service provides primary and preventive care, and during the COVID-19 pandemic it played a vital role in protecting Indigenous people living remotely in closed communities.

The need to be close to or on Country when dying means that the delivery of palliative services can only take place on a person's

Country; it is only there that their wellbeing is assured.[36] Purple House is the most innovative response to this need.

Sorry business can take weeks, and even months in some communities, which non-Indigenous people may not appreciate. Traditionally, the dwelling of the dead person would be burnt. Instances of this are now quite rare, though leaving the home for a 'sorry' camp is still common. The dead person's possessions were also burnt but are now more likely to be disbursed among relatives, the hope still being that the spirit does not come back. Ritualised self-harm can occur at funerals and was sometimes part of the social obligation; it was thought to help grieving and avoid mental anguish. A group of Elders, such as the Ngangkari, also perform a post-mortem assessment of the reason for death. This is as important to such Elders as a coroner's report is for non-Indigenous people. The death ceremony itself also varies depending on the circumstances and how far away from Country the family is living. Some have both a Christian and a traditional funeral, others in metropolitan areas are more likely to have Western funerals, and in many instances it is a combination of beliefs and traditions. Sharing food, singing and dancing are usual at most funerals.

Attendance at funerals is clearly important for Indigenous people in towns, regions or in remote communities. Given the high rates of death (including in young people from suicide and accidents), there is usually a funeral and sorry business every week in Perth. Workplaces need to accommodate the expectations of Indigenous people who are pulled to attend these ceremonies and have to take time off work. In an article on end-of-life ceremonial practices, Pam McGrath and Emma Phillips state: 'It is their right to mourn in a way appropriate to their culture, and our responsibility to show compassion and respect rather than bewilderment and misunderstanding.'[37]

The major message from this section on dying on Country is like that from the birthing stories. Culture is still alive, and although it may have adapted significantly, even in cities it can be very strong. To give First Nations people the way of dying that they want and need for their spiritual and cultural strength is really just a matter of asking and listening to them. While it may be challenging to provide palliative care on Country, it can be done in ways that are very healing for First Nations people. I was told of a woman who was dying of respiratory failure, and with family support the services managed to get her back on to her island. As there was no electricity, a small generator was installed so that she could receive her nasal oxygen and she was able to die peacefully on her land.

———

As a non-Indigenous person, I have found that obtaining the information for this chapter was quite riveting. The birthing symposium was one of the best meetings I have ever attended, and the more I read and interviewed people about birthing and dying, the more I realised how powerful, nurturing and caring these practices are. I would have loved to have birthed my two daughters with a doula and in a beautiful environment, to have buried their placentas in a special place that we could then have visited to heal and manage the spiritual aspects of our lives. I would not like to die in a large and busy hospital with people who are trying to keep me alive against all the odds. I would prefer to be at home with my family and die more naturally. For me the message is that both birthing and dying are part of our circle of life, they are not really medical conditions. We should look closely at these traditional Indigenous knowledges and take from them those aspects that would make our lives and life events so much more meaningful.

4

COMMUNITY CONTROL AND PRIMARY HEALTH CARE

SANDRA EADES

Growing up, I listened to my mother and other adults in my family talking about the health treatment they'd received during the difficult early years of their lives on the Gnowangerup mission. There was a doctor and a hospital at Gnowangerup but Aboriginal people who needed health care waited outside on the hospital's verandah. At the end of the day, when the doctor had finished seeing all the non-Aboriginal people who needed care, he would come out and see the Aboriginal patients who were sick. There was no birthing of Aboriginal babies at the hospital. Aboriginal babies were delivered by the Aboriginal midwife down at the Gnowangerup mission, where my mother was born in 1938.

Throughout the 1900s, Aboriginal people were increasingly moved off their traditional Country by the governments of the day and forced to live on missions or reserves, where they were racially segregated and separated from other Australians. Living conditions were poor and gave rise to many health problems that did not necessarily exist when Aboriginal people had freedom, living on their traditional lands.

I was born in 1967 and, as my birth certificate shows, I began my life living on the Mount Barker Native Reserve with other Noongar people and my family. In the decades before my birth, Aboriginal people like my mother, father, grandparents, aunties and uncles, could only move about off missions and reserves during the day to work; at night they could not be on the streets after six o'clock or sunset. The land allocated for missions and reserves where Aboriginal people lived was often of such poor quality that no one else wanted it. The Mount Barker Native Reserve was cold and damp, positioned between the town sewerage plant and a creek that ran alongside the railway line. This inferior land was not suitable for development and even today, although the native reserve no longer exists, it remains unused bushland, with some of the foundations of the old houses still there.

Our two-roomed house with its concrete floor, tin walls and a wood fire was also cold and damp, and with my mother, father, three brothers, sister and me all living there, it was overcrowded. There was no shower or toilet. The whole community had a shared communal shower and toilet block, again built with concrete floors and tin walls. There was also a community hall with wooden floors and tin walls. The poor living conditions and the stress of being segregated made life challenging in those years. I can recall an outbreak of tuberculosis in our region and the Western Australian Health Department coming to the reserve to screen everyone for TB. My brother Stafford and many other adults and children tested positive and needed to be treated in hospital in Perth for many months before they could come home again.

HEALTH CARE SELF-DETERMINATION VERSUS ASSIMILATION

I don't recall seeing a doctor during the years of segregation when we lived on the Mount Barker reserve. Once we moved into town in the early 1970s, I do remember seeing Dr Bourke, the town's doctor, in his consulting rooms, and going to the local hospital. My mother gave birth to all her seven children in the Mount Barker hospital, whereas her birth was a traditional one on Country in Gnowangerup.

Historian Anna Haebich writes about health politics and policies impacting on Noongar people during the early 1900s through to beyond the 1967 referendum.[1] She notes that the policy of assimilation had a major impact on Aboriginal health through the mid-20th century. For the first time, Australian governments endorsed the notion of equal citizenship for Aboriginal people, with full access to mainstream medical and hospital services, which had previously been denied to them. However, the transition to full access was contested and complicated by ongoing discrimination against Aboriginal people trying to receive health services. The government of Prime Minister Robert Menzies failed to adopt a policy of universal health insurance like Britain had done, and the lack of money to afford to pay for doctors' visits was an ongoing barrier to access for Aboriginal people, many of whom were living in poverty. In addition, Haebich notes the ongoing impact of poor living conditions, perpetuating poor health among Noongar people. David Thomas, in his PhD, 'Reading doctors' writing: Race, politics and power in Indigenous health research', notes that the way in which doctors wrote about Aboriginal people conveyed the notion that they were diseased and contagious and should not be allowed into spaces with the rest of the population for fear that infectious diseases such as hookworm could be transmitted to them.[2]

Haebich writes that my Noongar community had been devastated by the process of colonisation during the 1800s and an estimated population of between 6000 and 13,000 was reduced to 1400 by 1901. My ancestor Tommy King had thirty-four of his relatives die at one time because of a measles outbreak, so I can only imagine the distress of these years and the impact on Noongar people's mental and physical health. My grandparents and parents eked out a living working on rural farms during the 1900s, under the control of the Chief Protector of Aborigines AO Neville. They told stories of these times when Neville regulated every aspect of their lives. Letters in my mother's Native Welfare files outline the efforts my grandparents Muriel and Ivan went to, corresponding about their health needs, seeking permission to marry, or to buy shoes or move to another location. This level of oppression was hard and impacted on their health. Muriel and Ivan, who were loving and stoic people, both died young from heart disease and cancer. Clearly Noongar people suffered throughout the 1900s, and there was a need for leadership and action. They needed to shift from being passive subjects beholden to the will of colonial governments that were proposing assimilation as a new way forward for Noongar people – these people having failed to die out as many commentators, such as anthropologist Daisy Bates, believed they would.

In the 1920s, Noongar people struggled with these calls for assimilation. Haebich writes about the Noongar people's distrust of outsiders and authority and their readiness to stand up for their rights. Remember that at this time Indigenous people were not allowed to walk freely down the streets and, with a curfew in place, had to be off the streets by 6 pm. No wonder they were sceptical about the theory of assimilation. During and after the war, the hopes of Noongar soldiers, including my grandfather Sidney Eades and his brother Howard Eades along with others, were raised, their thinking being that fighting and contributing during the war would mean they were treated fairly and equally on their return home. Even the Returned Soldiers League backed Aboriginal ex-servicemen's claims for citizenship.

In 1947, The Coolbaroo League was established by Noongar people in Perth as an expression of cultural strength and unity. It was one of the earliest organisations set up by Aboriginal people for Aboriginal people. Aboriginal people were increasingly embracing self-determination, as opposed to assimilation, as an organising philosophy.

THE BEGINNINGS OF THE ABORIGINAL MEDICAL SERVICES

In the 1970s, there was a growing recognition of the need for self-determination and empowerment among Aboriginal communities. In Western Australia this was led out of the Aboriginal Advancement Council in Beaufort Street in East Perth, close to where many urban Noongars lived. The New Era Aboriginal Fellowship was formed to advocate for self-determination. This led to both the emergence of the Aboriginal community-controlled health movement and the WA Aboriginal Legal Service. These sought to empower communities to take control of their own health-care and legal services. The establishment of community-controlled health organisations, such as the Aboriginal Medical Services (AMS) and Aboriginal Community-Controlled Health Services (ACCHS), played a pivotal role in improving Aboriginal health. These organisations were founded on the principles of self-determination, cultural safety and community participation. They aimed to provide holistic, culturally appropriate health care that recognised the interconnections between physical, mental, emotional and spiritual wellbeing.

It was against this backdrop – and the 1967 referendum – that the first Aboriginal medical service was formed in Redfern in 1972. In 1973, three more Aboriginal medical services were established in Perth, Melbourne and Alice Springs. I am most familiar with the

Perth Aboriginal Medical Service (PAMS), having worked there as a high-school student on work experience in 1982 when I was fifteen years old. Initially unfunded and run by volunteers, by the time I went there as a student, the PAMS was well established. I later worked there as a young doctor in my twenties during the 1990s, and more recently as a member of the governing board in the 2020s. During these times, I met many of the legendary health leaders from my community – people who believed we should have control and be involved in providing health care to our mob and do a better job than mainstream services.

Apart from the doctors, all the other staff were Aboriginal. My grandfather Sidney Eades's cousin Aunty Joan Winch worked for the service as a community nurse. Aunty Joan was a well-loved figure at PAMS, visiting the many Noongar people who lived in Perth and East Perth in the 1980s. This was before the gentrification of these inner-city neighbourhoods. Aunty Joan knew that no Aboriginal people were being trained as health-care workers in Australian universities and colleges. It was also still very unusual for Aboriginal people to be trained in nursing or medicine at that time. She became a pioneer in the training of Aboriginal health workers in Western Australia, setting up her own college, Marr Mooditj ('good hands' in Noongar), to train an army of Aboriginal people who could provide health care in both AMSs and in mainstream services.

Joan Winch had visited China as a nurse in the early 1980s and was shown the 'barefoot doctor' program there. This was a pioneering system that was established throughout China during the 1960s and 70s, amid the political upheaval of the Cultural Revolution.

It provided a 'labour force' of people who received short-term training in medicine – anything from three to six months and up to two or three years. Although these people were not fully fledged doctors, they worked across the countryside in public health centres, with a focus on prevention.[3] After her visit to China, Aunty Joan Winch immediately realised the possibility of training such health professionals for our AMSs and adapted the barefoot doctor model to Western Australia. Marr Mooditj grew from strength to strength on very limited funding. It was recognised by the World Health Organisation in 1988 when it won the 'Nobel Prize' of public health, the Sasakawa Award, which included the sum of $40,000. This funding enabled Marr Mooditj to be even more successful.

Marr Mooditj students came from all over Western Australia to Perth to study at the school in Clontarf, which used to house Stolen Generations children. They had to have literacy and some numeracy skills, and they would receive four to five weeks of intensive lectures on all aspects of health and diagnosis and management of diseases. The students would then spend the rest of their time on Country with remote supervision to hone their skills and apply them to local conditions. Subsequently this model was successfully used to train Aboriginal health workers across the nation and at the Australian National University when it set up its Aboriginal Masters of Applied Epidemiology course. Thus, the impact of Joan Winch's vision has been enormously important for the primary health-care workforce in Australia and globally.

NATIONAL ABORIGINAL HEALTH STRATEGY, 1989

The *National Aboriginal Health Strategy* (NAHS), published in 1989, is an archival document that should be understood by anyone with an interest in the way in which Aboriginal communities engaged with state and territory and Commonwealth governments to lay the foundations for better health for future generations.[4] When I started work as a young doctor for the Perth Aboriginal Medical Service in the early 1990s, the NAHS provided a widely recognised new policy framework that shaped the delivery of health services.

Because it was such a landmark document, I would like to mention some of the other Aboriginal health leaders involved in writing the NAHS. We learn prominent names in history and too few of those named are Aboriginal. Naomi Mayers, a luminary in the early history of Aboriginal health and long-time CEO of the Redfern AMS, chaired the working party that oversaw the development of the health strategy, and my long-time friends Shane Houston and Ted Wilkes were members. Shane and Ted would contribute to many other aspects of Aboriginal health reform as well, including the NHMRC Research Roadmap and the Values and Ethics guidelines for Aboriginal health research. There were other Aboriginal leaders from every state and territory involved in writing the NAHS, as well as Aboriginal people working for state and territory governments and two Commonwealth government representatives.

I was fortunate to be able to meet and work alongside some of these early Aboriginal health leaders during the early years of my career. If you listened to them speak, much of what is reflected in the

NAHS was reinforced as critical to taking individual communities and linking them together in a national coalition, working in partnership with all levels of government to forge better health for Aboriginal people.

The NAHS laid the foundations for much of what has followed through the 1990s, 2000s, 2010s and the early 2020s. The health strategy document noted that in Aboriginal society there was no word, term or expression for 'health' as it is understood in Western society. It further explained: 'it would be difficult from the Aboriginal perception to conceptualise "health" as one aspect of life. The word as it is used in Western society almost defies translation, but the nearest translation would be a term such as "life is health is life".'

The connection between people with each other, with Creator Spirits and with the land, and an interdependence between the three, was highlighted and these connections resonated with what I was taught by my family growing up on Country and at key points during my life, including the birth of my son and the death of my mother.

The strategy emphasised that: 'Aboriginal spirituality was, and is, essentially land centred. Aboriginal people were totally dependent on the land and on all it could provide, and to benefit they developed social organisation that would enable them to use their natural environment successfully.'

The *National Aboriginal Health Strategy* also paid tribute to traditional Aboriginal health methods and contrasted them with Western health methods, which it noted were primarily interested in the recognition and treatment of disease. My experience in medical school was all about disease recognition and understanding pathways to refine and confirm diagnoses and institute appropriate evidence-based treatments. In contrast, Aboriginal medicine 'seeks to provide a meaningful explanation of illness and to respond to the personal, family, and community issues surrounding illness ... Aboriginal medicine and practices are a complex system closely linked to land based cultural beliefs and for this reason Aborigines in contemporary Australia see health as a sovereign issue.'

Many important definitions were provided in the *National Aboriginal Health Strategy*, such as this definition in its preface: 'This working party ... sees health as: Not just the physical well-being of the individual but the social, emotional, and cultural well-being of the whole community. This is a whole of life view and it also includes the cyclical concept of life-death-life.'[5]

I noted in my personal introduction how even today we are linked to our ancestors and my mother's passing brought us to a new phase of family life. We welcomed new great-grandchildren she would never meet, but who we would have the cultural responsibility to nurture and raise, without the confines of a nuclear family concept of life.

It's important to recognise that the NAHS was not anti-science, as this definition shows:

> Our working definition of primary care is: Essential health care based on practical, scientifically sound, socially and culturally acceptable methods and technology made universally accessible to individuals and families in the communities in which they live through their full participation at every stage of development in the spirit of self-reliance and self-determination.[6]

The NAHS definition of primary care welcomed new discoveries and showed that health care would evolve with these discoveries.

It also defined community control as 'the local community having control of issues that directly affect their community'. This was an important concept and a means by which Aboriginal people could counter the systems non-Aboriginal people imposed on them in relation to health.

During my career I have worked for Aboriginal community-controlled health services and served on the boards of these services. Every annual general meeting demonstrates the process of community control, as members of the community turn up to review their own service's progress in catering to the health needs of local Aboriginal people.

The NAHS also made some important and ground-breaking recommendations that shape the organisation and operation of Aboriginal primary care services today. It recommended the establishment of the National Aboriginal Community Controlled Health Organisation (NACCHO), as well as the establishment of the first committee to bring together representatives of NACCHO with state and territory and Commonwealth governments, to guide a unified community and government approach to all aspects of Aboriginal health improvement.

NATIONAL ABORIGINAL COMMUNITY CONTROLLED HEALTH ORGANISATION (NACCHO)

If I reflect on my career, there are many milestones important to Aboriginal health improvement. The establishment of the National Aboriginal Community Controlled Health Organisation is one of those milestones. NACCHO is a peak body representing Aboriginal community-controlled health organisations from around Australia. It was set up in 1992, the same year as Eddie Mabo's historic win in the High Court of Australia and Prime Minister Paul Keating's Redfern Speech. NACCHO took over from the National Aboriginal and Islander Health Organisation (NAIHO), which was itself established in 1975 by early Aboriginal health leaders.

As well as the 1989 release of the NAHS and the establishment of NACCHO, there were other important milestones. The 1987 Royal Commission into Aboriginal Deaths in Custody, and the release of the *Bringing Them Home* Report in 1997, on the separation of Aboriginal and Torres Strait Islander children from their families. I met Sir Ronald Wilson, the Chair of the enquiry, who invited me to join the panel, but I declined, feeling I wasn't able to listen to the anguish of personal stories I knew would be told around the country. Many of these stories I had heard while working as a GP in the Aboriginal Medical Service. The 2008 Apology to the Stolen Generations by Prime Minister Kevin Rudd and the launch of the first Close the Gap strategy were key to progress.

As contrast to these positive milestones, the 2014 budget of Prime Minister Tony Abbott and Treasurer Joe Hockey removed

$500 million dollars from Aboriginal programs, including many cultural and recreational programs not considered essential to Aboriginal wellbeing.[7] And yet culture and land are the basis of Aboriginal wellbeing. In 2018, the Coalition of Peaks (a national organisation of all the peak bodies for Aboriginal-controlled services) was established to get the Closing the Gap process for health back on track and foster the genuine engagement of Aboriginal communities. In 2023, a public communique by NACCHO reported being 'sure governments now see their national footprint of 550 plus clinics as providing a critical resource with which all organisations and agencies can partner. NACCHOs are accessed by 586,000 people each year and represent the largest employer of Aboriginal and Torres Strait Islander people in the country.'[8]

I feel fortunate to have witnessed many of the positive changes and, along with other Aboriginal health leaders, to have persevered when setbacks emerged. I stood in the Sydney Opera House and witnessed the sadness and disappointment of many in the audience when former Prime Minister John Howard refused to apologise to the Stolen Generations. The next day I marched for reconciliation with many thousands across the Sydney Harbour Bridge. I also witnessed the hope, joy and pride of Aboriginal people and other Australians when I travelled to Canberra to stand with crowds of people outside the national Parliament to hear the historic Apology to the Stolen Generations.

At the heart of Aboriginal primary care are ordinary Aboriginal and Torres Strait Islander people living out their culture and their links to family, community and Country.

DERBARL YERRIGAN HEALTH SERVICE: A SUCCESS STORY

We want to finish this chapter with the story of Derbarl Yerrigan, from its commencement in 1973, as the Perth Aboriginal Medical Service, with a staff of five, a budget of $100,000 and 400 patients. Today Derbarl Yerrigan, Noongar name for the Swan River, has a workforce of 158, of whom 59 per cent are Aboriginal staff, five being Indigenous doctors, and has an annual budget of $22.7 million and almost 20,000 patients.[9] It is the pride of the Perth Aboriginal community.

The health service grew out of the New Era Aboriginal Fellowship, which was formed in 1969 to drive the establishment of an Aboriginal medical service in Western Australia. One of our authors, Fiona Stanley, was a member of the New Era Aboriginal Fellowship and, along with other founding members, attended celebrations of the fiftieth anniversary of Derbarl Yerrigan in 2023.

They were first located in Beaufort Street in East Perth, and in 1998 they moved to the current, purpose-built facility in Wittenoom Street. The building was designed with strong Aboriginal consultation, and it is now a most important centre for health, wellbeing, culture, art and debate. It is a wonderful space; many of the 1998 staff, including me, painted wall tiles with lots of different designs that welcome you as you enter the reception.

Two other important Aboriginal organisations are close by: Yorgum Healing Services (children and families support) and Wungening Aboriginal Corporation, which provides alcohol and drug services, a homeless facility and care for people coming out of prison or detention. Having the health service close to these other social services creates an easily accessible hub for families for the range of services they need. Derbarl Yerrigan now has four metropolitan clinics – all busy and successful – in Midland, Maddington and Mirrabooka, as well as the East Perth centre. These locations are close to the main population centres for Aboriginal people in metropolitan Perth. The clients of the health service are not only Noongar families, as many urban-dwelling Aboriginal people from all over Western Australia come to it. The success of Derbarl Yerrigan has stimulated the establishment of twenty-three other Aboriginal community-controlled health services in Western Australia, ranging from the southwest (SWAMS) to the Kimberley in the north (KAMS, Broome, Derby, Beagle Bay, Balgo, Bidydanga, Fitzroy Crossing, Halls Creek, etc). Given the struggle for funds and the need for Aboriginal health professionals, this has been a remarkable achievement.

Derbarl Yerrigan runs four specialist clinics, STD diagnosis, cervical cancer screening, hepatitis C, and many other services. The attendance rates are very high and successful cures (for hepatitis C, for example) are far higher than those achieved in mainstream services. They now have mental-health accreditation, and in response to the increasing numbers of kids with developmental disorders, such as fetal alcohol spectrum disorders, they are seeking proper funding for their paediatric service. A high proportion of children going into juvenile detention have FASD, ADHD, intellectual disability and other early developmental problems.[10] It is vital that these children are assessed before being sentenced, as they will require special therapeutic services.

In 2023, Derbarl Yerrigan won the WACOSS Community Service award for their COVID-19 response to their community, and they were announced as the top GP service nationally for the Royal College of GPs. This is a phenomenal success for what started as a struggling vision for self-determination in health way back in 1973!

The clear message is that Aboriginal knowledges and ways of doing in primary care are essential to improve the outcomes for Aboriginal and Torres Strait Islanders. The birth and spread of Aboriginal community-controlled health services are vital for the continued reduction in poor health outcomes. While we do not (yet) have a Voice to Parliament, there is clear evidence that these services need to be supported and funded adequately. The NACCHO leadership, with the Coalition of Peaks, has been outstanding in pushing the national agenda.

5

INDIGENOUS PEOPLE AND HOSPITAL CARE

SHAWANA ANDREWS

This is a story of love and fear, and of wonder and knowing. It is a story that captures a time of change in a large metropolitan children's hospital from 1994 to 2000, reaching both back and forward for occasional context or retrospective detail. Offering an Aboriginal lens on the human experience of health care when there is a disjuncture in ways of knowing, being and doing. This story is also, inevitably, one of loss and sorrow.

When I started working at the Royal Children's Hospital in Melbourne in 1997, the children I worked with called me 'Aunty'. This term belied my junior role but demonstrated their respect and understanding of cultural ways. It was interesting to me that they wouldn't do this in the presence of non-Aboriginal staff. They somehow sensed that it was something that didn't fit. There was a lot that didn't 'fit' at the hospital. The children navigated the hospital system in their own insightful way, understanding the thresholds of the environment they were in and the limit to which they could express their cultural identities. Modifying their language and behaviour in front of non-Aboriginal hospital staff was a way to keep themselves safe.

In the early years at the hospital, I was supervised by the Aboriginal Hospital Liaison Officer, Angela Clarke, a Gunditjmara woman who would become a lifelong mentor to me and to a number of other Aboriginal women over the years. The Royal Children's Hospital, in 1997, was at a pivotal moment in time. The *Bringing Them Home* Report was tabled in the Australian Parliament on 26 May 1997. It was the outcome of the Human Rights and Equal Opportunity Commission's 1995–1997 National Inquiry into the Separation of Aboriginal and Torres Strait Islander Children from their Families.[1]

An academic framework of cultural safety developed by Māori nurse Dr Irihapeti Ramsden was also emerging then, placing the determination of safety with the service recipient and the expectation for change onto the service provider.[2] The Aboriginal community understood this concept well, as the need for feeling safe and culturally affirmed was something they had experienced in their own lives, and the work being done in the hospital system was addressing this very issue. Angela, having started in the Liaison Officer role three years earlier, was making changes to one of the largest hospitals in Australia. This provided a dynamic context in which to be working in a hospital for children.

This story is not about me, nor is it really about Angela (I don't think she would mind me saying that), although her leadership and visionary work are central to it. It is a story of the Koori community of Victoria, and that of all Aboriginal and Torres Strait Islander children, families and communities from across the country who have needed care at the Royal Children's Hospital in Melbourne. It is also the story of hospital care within the broader Australian health system, as many of the underlying issues told by way of the Royal Children's Hospital example are consistent across the national health and political landscape. Tertiary health care is highly specialised and is usually provided in a hospital setting, as distinct from primary health care, which is the collection of services and care provided to people universally and which is usually the first contact someone will have with the health system.

The experience of being in a space that does not speak to you, respond to you, recognise or understand you is difficult. It keeps you from yourself and doesn't allow you to connect with your own identity. This is a common experience for Aboriginal people in hospitals, which are, ironically, spaces where attention to wellbeing is the focus. Hospitals have never been places for Aboriginal people, meaning the encounters within them do not account for spirit and song, or being in culture and on Country. There is a feeling that culture and identity should be left at the front door. Throughout Australia's history, hospitals have done little to change the way in which they have understood, and provided for, the needs of Aboriginal people. Little attention, too, is afforded to the contribution of Indigenous knowledges to health care.

There is a record of Aboriginal people being subjected to a colonial 'logic of elimination'[3] through removal, confinement and assimilation. The Frontier Wars and widespread massacres sought to remove Aboriginal people not only through lethal violence but through the destruction of systems of knowledge that Aboriginal society is built on. Displacement on missions, the introduction of disease and controlled environments that prevented access to health care and the expression of culture confined bodies and souls. The government's assimilation policies from the 1950s to the mid 1970s were predicated on the belief that we were a 'dying race'. This led to the removal of Aboriginal children from their families under the Half Caste Act and the expectation that 'all persons of Aboriginal descent will choose to attain a similar manner and standard of living to that of other Australians and live as members of a single Australian community'.[4]

Consistent with the above, and beyond the Frontier Wars, prevention of access to health care for Aboriginal people has been a key feature of Australia's health-care system. This has applied to both Western and Aboriginal systems of health through exclusion from primary and tertiary health care, and forced removal, which has prevented people from sustaining their good health on Country and harvesting traditional medicines, as well as the disruption of knowledge transfer. Stories about the denial of medical attention, including for children and birthing mothers, or segregated care in wards or on hospital verandahs are common and exemplify the overt racism of the hospital system up until the 1970s. In more recent times there has been a greater focus on inclusion of Aboriginal people in health care, but overall Aboriginal people's relationships with hospitals remain fractured, with racism at the forefront, and where different ways of thinking about and addressing health are not generally embraced.

Dr Ian Wronski's 1980 report for the Health Commission of Victoria, *The Growth and Development of under 5 Aboriginal Children in Shepparton and Mooroopna*,[5] is credited as the catalyst for the development of the current statewide Aboriginal Hospital Liaison Officer (AHLO) Program.[6] The report instigated a number of initiatives that included a Ministerial Working Party into Aboriginal Health in Victoria that led to the establishment of the Aboriginal Health Unit, later to be known as the Koorie Health Unit, and a statewide Aboriginal Hospital Liaison Officer Program, which was launched in 1982.[7] The program was driven by Wotjobaluk man and Elder Uncle Kevin Coombs, who was Manager of the Koorie Health Unit. Uncle Kevin once said to me, 'Ideally, the successes of this work should put us all out of a job.' His vision was one where all Koori children and those from further afield would receive the right support and care when they needed it, without the barriers they once faced simply because they were Aboriginal. Uncle Kevin died during the writing of this book and his life was celebrated for everything that he achieved but above all, for the kind, caring and humble man he was.

The recognition of the need to address the structural barriers to enable better medical care and hospital services during these years signalled a significant change in the Aboriginal community's ability to obtain tertiary health care.[8] Coupled with the Victorian Aboriginal Health Service (VAHS),[9] established in 1973 as an Aboriginal community-controlled primary health-care organisation, a statewide network of liaison workers specifically tasked with easing the ways for Aboriginal people to receive treatment in hospitals was an important step. Interestingly, the Royal Children's Hospital did not take up the opportunity to have an Aboriginal Hospital Liaison Officer through the program until 1984.[10] Aunty Dr Sarah Berg remembers when the Koorie Health Unit approached the hospital: 'When [Uncle] Kevin and I first met with medical staff from RCH to tell them that they were going to be given funding for an AHLO position, the response was "Do we have to? We would much rather have an assistant pathologist"!'[11]

Angela Clarke was the fifth Aboriginal Hospital Liaison Officer for the Royal Children's Hospital and was in the role from 1994 until 2000, at which time she moved to the VicHealth Koori Health Research Unit (later to be known as Onemda) at the University of Melbourne. Angela's work toward structural change at the hospital was driven by a community development and public health approach and identified essential ways for improving care for Aboriginal children. These included respect and understanding of Aboriginal knowledges, collecting data and admission rates to know who was coming in and what their needs were, looking at the way in which the hospital was organised and being accountable for the way it operated, the quality of services for Aboriginal children, and improving the general care for Aboriginal families. Each of these areas required funding and strategic thinking by hospital leaders, who were generally unfamiliar with the needs of Aboriginal families and the structural barriers they faced. A lot of work had to take place to earn the trust of Aboriginal communities, who had little reason to trust the hospital system. The limitations of the Aboriginal Hospital Liaison Officer Program that were experienced in the beginning are much the same today. Creating organisational change while delivering a service is hefty work. Also, increasing people's access to services does not in itself guarantee they receive equitable or non-discriminatory care. Not feeling safe or culturally affirmed within a health service leaves people feeling uncomfortable and reluctant to return, which impacts on their health.[12]

In 1998, Sir Ronald Wilson presented the Royal Children's Hospital Grand Round, a presentation held regularly in the hospital for medical, nursing and allied health-care staff. He was invited by a staff member who had given evidence to the inquiry. Ron Wilson, president of the Human Rights and Equal Opportunity Commission[13] from 1990 until 1997, co-led the National Inquiry into the Separation of Aboriginal and Torres Strait Islander Children from their Families, with Aboriginal Social Justice Commissioner Mick Dodson. Culminating in the 700-page *Bringing Them Home* Report, the inquiry was another shift in Australian historical truth-telling, ten years after the Royal Commission into Aboriginal Deaths in Custody. It found that the Australian Government had driven a systematic attempt to destroy Aboriginal culture by the forced removal of Aboriginal children from their families. Ron Wilson's Grand Round at the hospital that day was part of the truth-telling and accountability work that supported a dialogue between hospital and community. This was a groundbreaking moment for the hospital and its willingness to accept responsibility for its role in Aboriginal child removal.

In a hospital for children, there are a number of things that become apparent when working with Aboriginal and Torres Strait Islander children and their families. The common experiences of poverty and overcrowded housing, for example, are important aspects of health to understand. But there are also less recognised considerations that are often overlooked or misconstrued, such as Aboriginal parenting and child-rearing practices, the importance of place for Aboriginal people as they navigate the health system, Aboriginal knowledge systems around health and wellbeing, and the Aboriginal kinship and governance structures that are at play. As key features for supporting Aboriginal wellbeing, particularly child health, it was these that Angela and our team needed to keep in sight to make improvements to the health systems.

Children would mostly come to the hospital with their mothers, aunties or grandmothers. Sometimes with all of the above. Fathers were present also, although less often, for many reasons. The overwhelming presence of women as carers and advocates for their children was obvious. They were holders of family and kinship knowledge, carers of children and Elders, and most often the decision makers for their child's care. Aboriginal women felt a strong need to protect their children as they negotiated the hospital system. This stems from a history of women's kinship relations having been disrupted through the forced removal of their children and the destruction of women's Laws.[14] Aboriginal women were very present for their children at the hospital, where they offered a counter-narrative of Aboriginal motherhood. Grandmothers' Law provided the laws related to pregnancy, birthing and breastfeeding, which we have written about more fully in chapter 3. What I saw at the hospital was the strength of Aboriginal women's knowledge and kinship – and I saw this in abundance, ranging from gathering community support for a family at a child's admission or discharge, to singing a child's spirit into the Dreaming at their passing.

On her arrival at the hospital in 1994, Angela worked toward a number of changes. Her first step was to extend on the work the previous Liaison Officer, Robynne Nelson, had done with an Aboriginal advisory committee to support an Aboriginal voice and provide a channel of communication between the community and the hospital. Angela further developed the Aboriginal Liaison Policy Advisory Committee with both hospital and Aboriginal community membership. The senior hospital staff representation on the committee was integral to making the hospital a culturally safe place; it was not good enough to simply find ways around the barriers, the aim was to remove them. The influence of senior staff helped to do this. The committee sometimes met at the Victorian Aboriginal Health Service and for some non-Aboriginal hospital staff this was the first time they had been in an Aboriginal organisation. I remember one non-Indigenous staff member saying it was the first time they had experienced being the minority.

Through the course of Angela's work, it became apparent that her isolation as a liaison officer would become a barrier in and of itself, as she aimed to make the hospital a culturally safe environment. With the support of the chief social worker, her immediate manager Jane Miller, Angela was able to build a small team to reduce the isolation and extend the work being done. She was also able to secure some space for both the team and the children and families; importantly this space was away from the busy wards. This was a particularly valuable step that would provide families with a place in which they could relax, be themselves and engage with the team safely. The space, first a room in the main hospital building and then a bigger area in a separate but connected building, was a game-changer. Initially named the 'Koori Room' and then reconceptualised as the Aboriginal Family Support Unit (the Unit), it introduced a new way of working together. Suddenly Aboriginal families using the Royal Children's Hospital had a place within it that was culturally affirming, changing the impact Angela and the team could have.[15]

The Unit slowly established itself in the hospital, and the children and families who used it worked to make it their own, with artwork, photos and posters. It became a place in which 'talk' could happen, in whatever language, without the listening ears of the ward and with the privacy needed to discuss things with the team, make phone calls and arrangements, and spend time with siblings or the patients. The Unit was the place where ideas about cultural safety within a hospital, as expressed by the families themselves, were generated. While some of these ideas addressed the socio-economic circumstances, many were drawn from Aboriginal knowledge systems and ways of knowing, being and doing as they relate to health and wellbeing.

Relationality is about connectedness. It is central to the way Aboriginal people relate to the world. The world is understood, and engaged in, according to our relationships with other people, animals and the natural and spiritual worlds. The obligations of kinship Law, or practices associated with care of the sacred body, or death and dying, are difficult to manage in a hospital that isn't set up for them and that isn't very flexible. The difference between Western and Aboriginal ways of knowing, being and doing was particularly apparent during these times, and it was Angela's role to negotiate the cultural boundaries. As a Gunditjmara woman of western Victoria, Angela was not able to know all the cultural practices of those she worked with; she did, however, put into practice principles that supported a voice for Aboriginal families, giving them control over making decisions. Challenging the many assumptions hospital staff made and the status quo of the hospital as a one-size-fits-all system by finding space for the respect and consideration of Aboriginal ways was hard work. Angela was clear in her expectation of the hospital:

> The work over the last four years has been constantly evolving and hopefully improving, with no doubt other dimensions to explore and improve on. Now with two full-time workers and another worker part-time, we are providing a service that our people are entitled to. We are able to identify areas of need and act on those suitably. We listen to what our families are telling us could be done better by the hospital and try to adapt the system accordingly.[16]

A shift in thinking of this kind was new and it played out in many ways across both policy and practice and where the institutional 'norms' were challenged. With the exception of emergencies, all medical procedures in Australian hospitals require consent by the patient, or in the case of children, by their parent or guardian. For many Aboriginal families the process of giving consent was not so straightforward. A 20-minute conversation with a consultant or surgeon did not equate to informed consent when a multitude of hospital barriers were present. There were interpreting barriers, with little to no availability of interpreters, literacy barriers and barriers due to the inability of surgeons to speak in plain language. Time and place were sometimes obstacles – this related to making sure the right people could be at the hospital at the right time, with often little time available to prepare for this – and there were also trust barriers. The hospital didn't adequately recognise the distinct impact any of these had on Aboriginal families and how they made it difficult for Aboriginal families to gain the information they required to make informed decisions about medical procedures for their children. By developing trusting relationships, and through good planning, the Unit was able to mitigate most of these barriers; this involved a significant investment of time, and sometimes the inflexible structures of the hospital would not bend.

The kinship system, which is not necessarily biological, also needed to be taken into account when consent was sought. Angela educated surgeons, patient-care coordinators, nursing unit managers and many others in ways to adapt their work to include a place for Indigenous knowledges and practices, enabling them to be given equal consideration to Western ways in health care. This would result in intense planning around consent, so that whole families could attend a briefing about the surgery prior to giving this consent. In some instances, the actual consent was not provided by parents but, in keeping with kinship laws, by grandparents, aunties or uncles, or community Elders. Sometimes the work involved in gaining consent required phone consultations with Elders and community members who were interstate. Surgeons made themselves available at times that suited the community to discuss the surgery and answer questions. And many questions arose. Remote community health centres, Aboriginal health workers, liaison officers in other hospitals and Aboriginal community-controlled health organisations were all part of a network that was called upon, in different ways at different times, to assist in the planning for some of these arrangements. This change in practice, and subsequent policy, was important to meet the needs of Aboriginal families, and it needed the understanding of hospital staff and decision makers.

Shifting a legacy of fear and distrust is a tough job, however, and comes at great risk when you are part of the community. One day, while on the ward, I received a message that there was a phone call for me from a regional Aboriginal organisation. I was advised that a mother was bringing her baby to the hospital in several weeks for a procedure. As was generally the case, the Aboriginal organisation could offer transport and support for the mother and child, and I confirmed that I would arrange accommodation for them in Melbourne. The mother was nervous and scared. I noted this and we got to work preparing for their arrival; this included checking the surgery and child's details in the system, speaking to the treating team, booking the accommodation, ringing the mother ahead of time to introduce ourselves and answer any questions she had, and all the while communicating with the Aboriginal organisation.

Despite this work, what transpired was a reflection of the broader state systems within which Aboriginal children and families (mothers in particular) are scrutinised, and how this adds to the complexities of their safety. The young mother arrived, and the surgery took place. It was not out of the ordinary but required some specialised surgery and, as with any procedure, was not without risk. The recovery took longer than expected and resulted in a longer hospital stay than anticipated. The mother was well supported over this time and was feeling happy that the surgery had been successful. Unfortunately, however, during this time she was evicted from her private rental property on the basis that she had been late in paying rent. This triggered a series of events that led to the arrival of a regional child protection team at the child's hospital ward one evening, with the purpose of removing the baby from the mother's custody. Homelessness was cited as the reason. Due to the work we had done with the treating team and ward staff, and the sound relationships Angela had fostered throughout the hospital, the nursing unit manager contacted Angela through the after-hours system. Angela headed into the hospital to find out what was going on. She was able to work with the nursing manager to ensure the child was not discharged from hospital care into the custody of the child protection team.

The story of this mother and her baby is both simple and complex. Simple because she was a mother who loved her baby and ensured he received the care he needed. Complex because she was an Aboriginal mother. Complex because she had feared the hospital owing to its legacy of child removal, but had been told it would be okay. The Aboriginal Family Support Unit, under Angela's leadership, worked closely with a number of Aboriginal organisations to find housing for the mother. The nursing unit manager was able to extend the child's hospital admission until the family's accommodation was secure. Some time after the child's discharge home with his mother, however, we learnt that he had been removed from her care by Child Protection and placed in the care of a non-Aboriginal relative.

Hospitals are strange places. They are places where people are unwell or injured and where emotions are high. They are the workplaces of the 'caring' professions and usually promote values of respect and integrity. Yet they are not places that have much time for culturally diverse understandings of health or the wonders of the spirit and ancient practices of healing. The numbers and data generated within and by hospitals do not speak of these things. They speak of average length of stay, discharge rates, failure to attend, outpatient attendance, inpatient admissions and more besides. Aboriginal patients often rate worse than their non-Aboriginal counterparts on all such measures, but there is always a story behind the numbers.

When someone doesn't turn up for a hospital appointment, this is what is referred to as 'failure to attend'. At the Royal Children's Hospital, we knew that this was a big problem and we knew why. The value of having Aboriginal people working in a hospital and having a safe place within it underlined the worries some Aboriginal parents face. There were issues such as transport and money worries that sometimes prevented some families from coming to the hospital, but the biggest concern was how some Aboriginal families felt they were being judged. Aboriginal parenting and the way we grow up our children is grounded in kinship, where parenting is often shared, and aunties are mothers and uncles are fathers. The concept of family is rarely built on the nuclear family model and the way we see our children is often fundamentally different. The Aboriginal model generally trusts the child's knowing which adults are obliged to respond to.[17] Babies and children are generally supported to live in relation to people and the world around them, which means their place in family and community is set, along with all the responsibilities of Law and culture.

Elders and grandparents have a central place and often have decision-making roles, and child-rearing practices reflect the importance of developing independence and resilience in children. Children are given the freedom to explore the world around them and are part of cultural and spiritual teachings that help them know who they are, and where and how they belong. However, Aboriginal parenting has been targeted in assimilation policies in the past and continues to be besieged by current state child removal practices.[18]

It is important for children to attend their appointments. By putting in place one essential practice, Angela and our team were able to reduce the failure to attend rate to less than 10 per cent. In the days leading up to an appointment, we would call the family to remind them of their appointment, ensure they had a way to get there and let them know we would meet them. The creation of trusting relationships with patients in this way significantly improved attendance and showed that Aboriginal ways of knowing, being and doing were possible in the hospital system. In 1999, we wrote a book called *Lookin' After Our Own*[19] to try to capture what the Aboriginal Family Support Unit was doing to change the hospital.

The experience of being in hospital is a complex one. The nature of disadvantage that Aboriginal communities live with as a result of colonisation necessitates a high use of tertiary health care. In the previous chapter, we explored how Aboriginal communities have built an effective primary health model that is based within community; hospitals are yet to achieve anything similar. We are seeing much good work happening in hospitals across Australia though, and Aboriginal knowledges are starting to be recognised and accepted. Possum skin cloaks have a role in healing in some hospitals, traditional healers such as the Ngangkari have a hospital role in some places, and smoking ceremonies and other ways to honour the sacred body are now sometimes accepted. But there are still high levels of racism[20] and ineffective care across the health system. Angela's work at the hospital is similar to that of many Aboriginal Hospital Liaison Officers around the country, all working to bring Aboriginal knowledges into view so that hospitals can better understand how to deliver their services. The work done at the Royal Children's Hospital during this time and beyond saw much change, but the work of a few Aboriginal strategists in such large dynamic organisations is like a drop in the ocean, especially when doing it against the tide. The continuity of the work and its sustained impact is easily lost when there is no senior advocacy or drive.

Angela has now returned to her Dreaming and is with her ancestors, but her work endures and those of us who benefited from knowing her keep her close to our hearts. Every now and then I will meet someone who brought a child to the hospital during those years and they'll say to me, 'She was good that one. What was that liaison officer's name there, Angela hey?'

6

TRADITIONAL LIFE FOR HEALTH

SANDRA EADES

Have you ever looked at photographs or drawings of Aboriginal people at the time of first contact and early contact with British settlers? Photos of my ancestors, the Minang Noongars from the Albany region of Western Australia, show that both men and women are lean and muscular with very little or no body fat. Compared to life then, life now shows that being overweight or obese is very common among Aboriginal children and adults and people of other ancestry in most regions of Australia.

Despite the fact that we were dispossessed of our traditional lands, we can learn from the health and lifestyle of our ancestors.

We can consider how we can apply what we learn to the way we live today to help us stay lean, fit and healthy.

My ancestor Wandinyilmernong, or Tommy King, made the first written Australian land claim in a petition written for him by colonisers at the time of the celebration of the granting of self-government to the Western Australian colony.[1] Tommy King's petition from October 1890 noted that Albany rightly belonged to his people and had been stolen by agents of the British Crown. A consequence of this land theft was his people being deprived of their dignity and their means of making a living. Noongar people had to struggle to adapt to the impact of colonisation. They were forbidden access to their land with its bounty of traditional foods and the freedom to walk and hunt, guided by the six Noongar seasons. As well, some were working long hours for limited pay, while still trying to collect and prepare food from traditional sources every day, as their access to food from the colony was limited.

YEARLY CYCLES FOR THE NOONGAR PEOPLE

Growing up living on Noongar boodja (land) in the far southwest of Western Australia, I lived in a small country town close to the ancestral lands of my Minang Noongar people. From Albany to Bremer Bay, inland to Gnowangerup and the sacred Toolbroonup ranges, then across to Kojonup, Cranbrook and the Frankland River areas were the places and lands of my ancestors. Albany is known by Noongar as Kinjarling or 'place of rain', and settlers were to name Toolbroonup the Stirling Ranges.

Life for Noongar was cyclical, and those cycles ran through each calendar year and their seasons. The cycles also ran through the years of each person's life and their particular roles and responsibilities in the family over their lifetime. Babies were born near their birthing tree with mothers supported by their own mother and grandmother. Joining the family in the main camp several weeks after birth, life continued for each new baby and koolungar, young children. Young people learned their responsibilities and later married someone who was seen as appropriate according to families and through our contemporary understanding of historic skin groups. Throughout life, our responsibilities to our families continue even in contemporary times.

The Noongar calendar has six seasons. Birak (December and January), Bunuru (February and March), Djeren (April to May), Makaru (June to July), Djilba (August and September) and Kambarang (October and November). These seasons and the change in plants and animals grounded our family and community life on Minang Noongar boodja. Health was incidental to life. Exercise did not need to be programmed; it was part of the process of living. Life on Country, socialising, relational being – one's way of being in relation to family, kin and Country – hunting and gathering, and preparing and eating food produced lean, healthy looking, muscular people, and good mental health for groups of people and individuals. In some historical records we are known for our activity as firestick farmers and yonga (kangaroo) pastoralists and for our use of ingenious weirs for taking fish in the King George Sound at Albany.[2]

BIRAK, DECEMBER AND JANUARY

Birak is the Noongar season running from December to January. The rain disappears and the hot weather intensifies. Hot easterlies blow in the morning and cool breezes off the sea appear in the afternoon. Traditionally, this was fire season and Noongar would burn the Country in mosaic patterns. The land depended on fire to regenerate the bush and allow for new growth of sweet grasses that attracted the yonga after the first rains of the season. There are many fledgling birds out in nests in Birak, such as parrots and magpies. Snakes and bobtail, bluetongue and other lizards are shedding their skin.

Further south from Perth I recall my grandfather Sidney Eades would burn the 44 acres of land across the road from his house. My grandfather's careful firestick burning of this land on the outskirts of Cranbrook in the 1970s was a practice he learned from his family, cultivating a pristine landscape clear of heavy undergrowth for us to play in as koolungar, kids.

BUNURU, FEBRUARY AND MARCH

Bunuru, in February and March, is the hottest time of the year. Hot easterly winds regularly blow, and in the afternoons comes the cooling sea breeze close to the coast. Traditionally, this was a good time to be living near the coast, fishing and eating crustaceans like gilgie and garon, and fishing for mullet in the river near Bremer Bay and Albany. Our family would camp by the ocean and spend whole days out on the land or by the sea, fishing and being together.

We would travel to places by the coast that our family had visited seasonally over millennia. We would go to large inland lakes and be taught to swim surrounded by family, giving us confidence to go out into the water and copy older siblings or cousins – learning by seeing and doing. At times we would get hurt, be bitten by an ant, or fall over and scrape our skin. Older members of our family knew what bush medicines or remedies to use to treat those hurts. A common plant along the coast is coastal pigface and the fruit is edible and the succulent leaves can be broken open like aloe vera to rub on skin rashes or other hurts.[3]

Bunuru is also the time of gums including jarrah and marri that grow in abundance to flower, and the time when the manna gum tree (manna wattle) sheds clear white gum from its trunk.[4] We would walk for miles around the bush tracks on our traditional lands that surrounded the towns where we now lived. Sometimes we were looking for manna gum or we would walk creeks and dams to look for gilgies to catch and eat. You could tell a gilgie burrow in a creek as it piled mounds of mud up around the outside of where it had burrowed deep in the soft waterlogged soil at the edge of the water. My brothers would put their hands down the burrow, sometimes up to their elbow, and be djerpin, happy, whenever they pulled out a fresh live gilgie. Gilgie was one of the sweetest feeds we could catch even as kids.

Any time we had free was spent outdoors in the bush or camping out with family, walking trails and listening to Elders and older siblings and cousins. Sometimes we walked across fenced fields and pastures and were chased by new landowners on horses or motorbikes, telling us to get off their land. We didn't realise at the time that we were experiencing the ongoing impacts of colonisation and invasion, where we were forcibly removed from our ancestral lands that support and nurture our lives.

DJEREN, APRIL AND MAY

Djeren comes in April and May. Djeren sees a break in the hot weather, with cooler nights and dew on the ground in the mornings. The winds change their direction, with light breezes blowing up from the south. Growing up, we would walk across Country, especially a week or so after the first rains, looking for mushrooms that would spring up in the forest and paddocks.[5] Mushrooms were prolific and we could easily eat a plateful after a day or afternoon of walking and looking for raised clumps of soil where the mushrooms peeked up through the earth. Outside of Melbourne, where I now live most of the year, I like to go looking for mushrooms in the autumn and I am reminded of time collecting field mushrooms with my parents and grandparents – being taught the difference between a mushroom that was safe and edible and those that were not safe to eat.

MAKARU, JUNE AND JULY

Makaru comes in June and July and brings rain and colder weather. Makaru is the coldest and wettest time of the year, and it was good to be farther from the coast then, away from the stronger southerly and westerly winds that bring large amounts of rain.

HEALTH

As the streams and creeks filled with water, people could live further inland and hunt yonga. I remember the streams running and even underground water coming up from the ground in springs where we lived. Sometimes in the deepest, coldest part of the year it snowed on Bulla Meeyle, the highest point in the sacred Toolbroonup hills. Bulla Meeyle was called 'Place of many faces and eyes' and was a place where the ancestors went to rest. Your 'eyes' are your meeyle in Noongar and bulla is 'many' in Noongar. While we would often go to these sacred ranges during the day to walk with family, we would make sure we were gone by sunset, as these were very spiritual places where the Pullyit spirits were, and people should not be there after dark. If you were stuck and unable to leave before dark or sunset, you needed to light fires to keep the Pullyit away. Many stories are told of the Pullyit at Toolbroonup and why to stay away at dark.

My mother's brothers would hunt and catch the native duck in this area for food. It was a lot of work to prepare the duck for eating, but we would have a great feast when we could find them. Both my mother's and father's families would hunt for yonga, kangaroo, a traditional source of food. My eldest brother also recalls our Elders cleaning and curing the yonga skin to make a booka, cloak, for warmth when he was young. Finding yonga involved walking long distances through the bush late in the day or early in the morning when they grazed. The rhythms of life required effort, and a lot of time was spent moving and walking together as a group to hunt or fish or go from one place to another.

As we played, we made pretend mia mia in the bush from branches and leaves, building our own little camping places with these shelters and fires. It was a lot of work to make your camp. Even though we drove, we would get out of the car and walk to be on Country and to go to the place in the bush where we could swim or camp or walk to a creek to get gilgies or when hunting for yonga. My grandfather Sidney once took all of us hunting for yonga – we were able to get to our initial destination by car but then we needed to go by foot to make enough noise for the kangaroo to start moving in the evening. We would also drive out to get firewood, walking through the bush to collect it and taking it home for the outside fire. As well as the wood fire inside the house, Pop Sidney always had the outside fire burning in the colder months of the year.

My mother, who was born in 1938, recalls as a young woman walking about 20 to 30 kilometres cross country on most Friday afternoons, from the farm where her family lived at Beejenup to the town of Broomehill, to visit her grandmother and cousins. We would walk long distances to see our relations and keep connected with kin. In earlier times, we would walk long distances to meet and trade with other clans of Noongars, exchanging ochre, the Kodja stone axe or other handmade implements. My father Stafford was born in Kojonup, a town named after the well-known Kodja or Noongar stone axe. On Sunday afternoon my mother and her sisters would walk back across Country to be home for work on Monday. They knew the paths to travel and copied the ancient ways of their ancestors, walking long distances across Country.

In late Makaru after much rain, the boronia begins to flower in the swamps and creeks fill with water. My grandmother and mother knew where to walk and find the boronia when in season. The wild potato could also be found and was recognised by a long green stem. The larger the stem, the larger the wild tuber buried in the ground, waterlogged and tasting bland and starchy. We would find a digging stick and go into the bush across the road from our house and spend many hours walking and digging up the wild potato to eat.

DJILBA, AUGUST AND SEPTEMBER

Djilba is from August to September and a time when the landscape bursts into flower, particularly far south around the ranges and forests and towns north of Albany, where we lived in the 1970s. When I was young, I thought the whole world had native flowers like the ones we grew up with, which would bloom in Djilba. I realised when I was older how ancient the landscape was and how rare these spring plants were in Australia and the world.

Warmer days are mixed with colder days and more rain at this time. The bush is alive and full of colour. On the warm days, you can walk for miles looking for the sweet mulberries and trawl through creeks and dams looking for gilgies again as the weather warms. Traditionally food came from yonga, waitch (emu) and koomal (possum). To find waitch or waitch eggs on the plains or to hunt yonga took time to walk, follow subtle signs and know where to look. These animals graze with their young and take care of them. The woodlands are full of birds and their offspring including koolbardi (magpie), chitty chitty (willy wagtail) and chuck-a-luck (wattlebird).

KAMBARANG, OCTOBER AND NOVEMBER

Kambarang comes in October and November. The days are warmer and there is an abundance of flowers – the acacia and banksia and smaller yonga (kangaroo) paws and orchids. All around the southwest, the moojar or Australian Christmas tree is on display with its bright yellow orange flowers. Koolbardies swoop to protect their young in the nest and snakes begin to move around, coming out of their winter hibernation. The bush is alive and small berries such as cumacs (small fruit) and manna gum can be collected while walking in the bush. One of our favourite pastimes was to walk through the bush collecting mulls during October – tiny green berries that grew on what is commonly known as the kick bush.[6] Our version of the 'kick bush' grew along the ground like a flat groundcover and the flowers were white.

TRADITIONAL ABORIGINAL WAYS OF LIFE MIRRORED IN MODERN HEALTH ADVICE

In Western medicine, exercise is now prescribed quite separately to pills because of its beneficial effect on health,[7] just as a diet rich in fruit, vegetables, lean meat, nuts and fish is beneficial. Spending time in nature is also recognised as important for good mental health. These principles are fostered around the world and modern humans find ways to maintain these practices for healthy lives.

In the traditional Noongar way of life that I partly experienced in my early years, exercise and diet and time in nature were not prescribed but were part of a way of being, where life was medicine and medicine was life. We were always active and moving, taking time and effort to find food and be in relation to family and on Country. Living within the movement of seasons and life and being with kin on Country were powerful and full of the medicine of life.

It is well established that outdoor, nature-based interventions improve mental health in individuals.[8] Time in nature reduces depressive symptoms, anxiety and negative moods, and improves positive moods. When we speak about time in nature, that description includes forest therapies and wilderness therapies, with an emphasis on immersion in nature for between four and eight weeks. Time in nature in a contemporary sense also includes gardening, especially over long periods of time and across seasons. I can only imagine the impact of losing access to one's Country and being removed from a lifestyle that was built on time in nature and shared with large groups of people, that sustained and nurtured Indigenous people's mental health. In the future, more efforts to reconnect with land and culture are certain to bring mental-health benefits to Indigenous people and reaffirm the importance of our connection to Country over tens of thousands of years.

PROFESSOR KERIN O'DEA'S STUDY OF THE HEALTH BENEFITS OF CHANGE FROM URBAN LIFE TO TRADITIONAL LIFESTYLE AND DIET

In a unique study at the time, Kerin O'Dea partnered with ten middle-aged Aboriginal men living with diabetes from the

Mowanjum community in northwestern Australia. The 1980s study sought to understand whether going out bush and living a more traditional Aboriginal lifestyle with camping and hunting can reverse some of the body's tendency to develop diabetes.[9] The men undertook a blood test before and after seven weeks of living as close as possible to a hunter-gatherer lifestyle, with a diet that was low in calories (1200 kcalories/person/day on average) and low in fat (because of the low-fat content of the animals hunted and eaten, and that fat being healthier than the fat found in beef cattle and sheep). Fasting and post-meal glucose, insulin and lipids were measured in the periods before and after the men reverted to their traditional Aboriginal lifestyles.

The tendency to develop diabetes was either greatly improved or completely normalised after this short period of camping and hunting to source food over several weeks. Three key factors – a weight loss of 8 kilograms on average, a low-fat diet and higher levels of physical activity – contributed to the changes in health. In carrying out this study, Professor Kerin O'Dea developed important relationships and trust with Aboriginal people and communities. They supported the work she was doing to demonstrate the beneficial health impact of Indigenous knowledges. She became a champion of traditional ways of living and any other contemporary adaptations to draw the benefits of traditional lives.

I was fortunate to be mentored by Professor O'Dea later in my life and career. I was always fascinated by her studies and our discussions about the nutritional benefits of traditional Aboriginal diets and lifestyle. Other Western researchers using other ways to accumulate and record knowledge were able to confirm what was known through Indigenous Australian knowledge systems about the benefits to physical and mental health stemming from Indigenous ways of life walking Country and living on Country.

PHYSICAL ACTIVITY AND EXERCISE RECOMMENDATIONS

The philosopher Plato wrote that 'Lack of activity destroys the good condition of every human being while movement and methodical physical exercise save it and preserve it'. Our ancestors would tell us the same, I am sure, with their knowledge of wellbeing built up through experience over thousands of years living on Country in this vast land.

My professional training and my Indigenous knowledge from growing up on Country show the importance of physical activity for health. Being physically active is not just about exercise and running on a treadmill, but about the relationship between humans and their environment. It is about using the body in the way it was designed to be used, to run sometimes, walk often and exert ourselves regularly, whether we are at home, work, school or doing things with our free time. Our ancestors knew this and the life I experienced growing up, living on Country with my parents and grandparents, aunties and uncles and cousins, was embedded in this ancestral knowledge.

My training in Western medicine reinforced the important lessons I had learned as a young person from my ancestors on Country. I understand the links between physical activity in a

Noongar way of life and health and, conversely, the major role a lack of physical activity plays in the development of heart disease and stroke, diabetes, obesity and some cancers, poor skeletal health, some aspects of mental health, and overall risk of dying, as well as poor quality of life. Men and women of all ages, socio-economic groups and ethnicities are healthier if they achieve the public health recommendation of at least 150 minutes per week of moderate-intensity aerobic physical activity, such as brisk walking.[10]

As I have noted in the early part of this chapter, being active and doing things such as walking, swimming, hunting and fishing as well as wood collection and fire-making all took physical effort. Our traditional lives were full of physical activity and exercise that was conducive to good health. We did not sit for many hours a day watching TV or playing computer games or reading our phones, text messaging and on social media. We were active and busy people who had many things to do just to manage eating and caring for ourselves.

CREATING THE CONDITIONS FOR INDIGENOUS PEOPLE TO STAY PHYSICALLY ACTIVE

While I have fond memories of growing up being physically active and on Country, that is not a reality for many Aboriginal people. We are too often restricted by poverty, living in poor community settings that don't support exercise and being physically active. In all our efforts to close the gap, we must be mindful that helping individuals and communities to stay physically active is as important to our future health as reducing the level of tobacco smoking. While the tobacco message has been taken up, with millions of dollars spent on programs to reduce smoking, efforts to improve opportunities for our communities to remain active and healthy are missing. Many sports and recreation clubs that support Aboriginal children, youth and adults to stay active are viewed as optional programs and not embedded in social and health policy to close the gap in health. Organisations such as the Rumbalara Football and Netball Club, run by the Aboriginal community in Shepparton, Victoria, to support participation in sport that is culturally safe and free of racism are as important to health as the local primary health-care clinic. Measures included in the Noongar Native Title settlement to secure land that will be handed back to Noongar communities will mean people can go on Country and once again be able to pursue cultural activities on Country. These activities are essential to supporting healthy, active lifestyles that were so common in traditional Indigenous ways of life.

Job opportunities that involve being on Country and caring for Country are integral to our future health. As Aboriginal people, we must be creative and draw on the strength of our ancestors' way of life as much as other aspects of life. We must support the next generation of young Indigenous Australians to rediscover Country and to be active and in nature, like our ancestors, as a way of achieving good health.

7

HEALTH AND CULTURAL PRACTICE

SHAWANA ANDREWS

In 2022, I had the good fortune to attend the Garma Festival, an Indigenous cultural exchange event hosted by the Gumatj clan at Gulkula. It's a celebration of the cultural, intellectual and ceremonial traditions of the Yolŋu people in Northeast Arnhem Land, shared with leaders who come from across the country to discuss the most pressing issues facing Indigenous communities. There on Gumatj Country, put on full display for those attending, I watched the buŋgal each day – the ceremonial dance and song that embodies intricate stories of Yolŋu life, histories and places. Buŋgal, with its elaborate painted visuals and red dust flying up around the feet of the dancers, has not been lost or dormant. It has survived colonisation and remains strong:

> To the Yolngu, our songs, paintings and dances are our books – they tell us where we have come from and where we are going to. They follow the songlines that weave us together. They are our maps, our law books, our title deeds, and our family history. They connect us to the land and the animals with which we share it and of whom we are a part. They are woven into our hearts.[1]

Cultural practices draw on archives of knowledge that are deeply embedded in Country and are maintained across generations, time and place. It is the linking of such places of significance that form the Songlines people travel to activate culture. As knowledge transfer occurs across the generations, the knowledge is refined, adjusted and cared for in response to generational changes, thus keeping them alive. Culture is dynamic and responsive, allowing it to shape-shift according to changing conditions. Practices can become lost through violent prohibition and destruction, or lie dormant for their protection and later reactivation. Contemporary expressions of Indigenous resilience and resistance can be seen in the resurgence of cultural ways, which are being reawakened across many facets of our lives. Aunty Joy Murphy, senior Wurundjeri Elder in Victoria, has worked tirelessly to support this work and her books *Welcome to Country* and *Wilam: A Birrarung Story*, beautifully illustrated by Lisa Kennedy, teach of Country, kinship, language, religion and economy, all of which have been identified as rich repositories for restoring knowledges that in turn enhance positive identity and wellness.[2]

There is an understanding that we must retain our culture for our health and futures. The possum skin cloak is an example of such revitalisation. If you lived in the southeastern parts of the continent, on the lands of the Kulin Nation perhaps, you would particularly value your possum skin cloak in Waring (wombat season, from April to July). Misty mornings are followed by cool days. It is the time of highest rainfall and lowest temperatures and is when waring venture out to bask and graze in the sunshine. Days become shorter and nights longer, and as the cold wind bites, you might pull your possum skin cloak closer around your shoulders. Much more than a source of warmth and comfort, the cloak would be etched, using shell or bone, with iconography of Country and designs of totems and kinship, making the cloaks themselves important repositories of knowledge, and imbuing the wearer with identity and belonging.

Yoolongteeyt Aunty Dr Vicki Couzens is a Gunditjmara Keerray Woorroong woman and a Senior Knowledge Holder for Possum Skin Cloak Story. Her work, along with others, in revitalising possum skin cloak making over the last thirty years has been instrumental in reinstating the practice as a means of supporting identity and healing. When Aboriginal peoples of southeastern Australia were dispossessed from their Country, they were provided with meagre food rations on government-controlled missions, and possum skin cloaks were replaced by inadequate blankets that harboured disease.

In a project I conducted in 2018, Yoolongteeyt Aunty Vicki taught me and a group of Aboriginal women how to make a cloak.

It was a project exploring women's experiences of family violence and the cloaking supported the women to tell their story. Importantly, the process helped them to engage with a practice many of them had never tried before and to own a cloak for their personal use. They used the cloaks for their babies and grandchildren, one was used in a palliative care setting, and others used it to learn about their totems so they could include them in the design. The project also provided a setting for the women to connect with one another in their healing and to understand their experiences of family violence. One woman said, 'For a lot of us that have never been in it [culture] this brings us back to who we really are and it gives us a sense of belonging, to being there.' And another said, 'You're more likely to be open that it was at a family violence group, because you're proud of the possum skin that you've made.'[3] Aunty Gina Bundle was also a part of this project and took photos of the women in their cloaks. The photos of these and many others that Aunty Gina has gone on to make, such as the Victorian Treaty possum skin cloak, have helped to share this experience. Reconnecting with and preserving knowledge in this way supports selfhood and identity.

Our Elders say that culture is Law, the foundation of the Indigenous world. The colonial damage – and in some cases decimation – of our cultural ways and systems of knowledge has contributed to a fractured cultural identity for many Indigenous peoples. Cultural identity is closely associated with cultural continuity, which is preserving our cultural traditions and carrying them forward into the future.

In groundbreaking work, Canadian researchers Chandler and Lalonde established that the restoration of cultural practices,

HEALTH AND CULTURAL PRACTICE

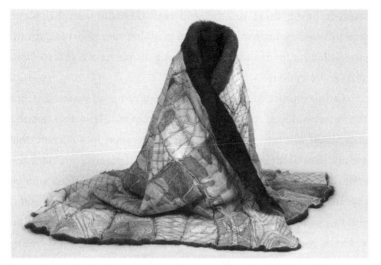

Reproduction of a Gunditjmara possum skin cloak collected in 1872 from Lake Condah, 2002 by Debra Couzens and Vicki Couzens, Gunditjmara/Keerray Woorroong people.

and the Indigenous knowledges that inform them, could act as protectors of health.[4] Resilience, agency and governance feature in their work toward the prevention of Indigenous youth suicide, and a number of important factors were identified that provided the right environment for cultural continuity. These pointed to things such as self-governance, access to education and land autonomy (i.e., treaty). The role of language is of particular note in their work. Chandler and Lalonde argue that each of these variables combine to create the circumstances that enable young people to build their identities on a cultural basis, without which self-destructive and suicidal behaviours manifest.[5] Across our communities, significant work is being done to find and reawaken our cultural ways; sometimes they have not been lost, in which case effort is put into strengthening them and ensuring young people have access to them and can learn them.

Cultural practice can be seen as the pouring of water. It is not the vessel holding the water, nor the recipient. It is also not the water itself, but rather the very act of conveyance. Its value and role are not simply functional, however – cultural practice provides the connectedness between the everyday and the systems of knowledge that inform it. Our ways of expressing culture can at once be useful and sacred, bringing to life Aboriginal worlds. If we think of culture as health, then its rituals, customs and traditions are central to health and wellness, connecting our everyday lives with the sacred teachings of our ancestors, giving us identity, purpose and belonging, and keeping us whole. The widespread revitalised possum skin cloaking practice, for example, now supports the wellbeing of people in areas such as family violence, palliative care, acute care and the engagement of young people.

In 2022, Professor Sandra Eades invited Professor Joseph Gone of Harvard University to Naarm (Melbourne) for a visit, during which he discussed the idea of 'culture as treatment'.[6] A member of the Aaniiih-Gros Ventre tribal nation of Montana in the United States, Professor Gone spoke in his lecture about the work he was doing to address substance use in Indigenous communities in the US. He focused on the role culture and its practices play in addressing significant substance use and associated health issues in Indigenous communities. A leading psychologist, Professor Gone says that 'the hope and promise of healing from addictions for Indigenous people are rooted in cultural interventions'.[7] It is within the ethos of connectedness and interdependence that Professor Gone and Indigenous Elders from around the world reframe health as wellness. This carries with it the understanding that while we manage the personal health problems that arise from the colonial experience, we must also focus on the challenges we face for achieving communal wellness, which requires 'bigger' thinking, for example treaty, or the power a voice gives to make policy decisions in health.

Culture and its constituent practices, such as ritual, ceremony and protocols, are by definition shared socially. They hold within them the link between present and future health across systems of kinship, language, religion and economy. Together they form an important scaffold for social and cultural wellbeing.[8] Health is an intrinsic part of the relatedness, belonging and continuity that comes from participating in ritual and ceremony and from following protocols, sometimes in the most subtle and refined but important ways. I have a precious maireener shell (or rainbow kelp shell) necklace made by Aunty Lola Greeno. Aunty Lola is a Pairrebeenne/Trawlwoolway Elder and shell artist and uses her art to connect an ancient practice to contemporary communities. Born on Cape Barren Island, Aunty Lola, like many shell stringers, was taught the practice by her mother and grandmother. She now shares this tradition with others, teaching and promoting the stories of Sea Country and the skill of collecting and stringing shells.[9] Shell stringing practice, kanalaritja, has been unbroken for Aboriginal women of Trouwerner (Tasmania), offering the practice of their ancestors to future generations.

Although many contemporary shell necklace makers once lived on the Furneaux Islands, most were pressured to leave the islands under the threat of child removal and so they could have better access to health services and education. This brought about significant social change that saw only a few surviving makers creating new work and sharing their skills and stories. The island women kept a tight hold on their knowledge about where to collect the shells and how to prepare them when making necklaces. This knowledge was, and still is, guarded information, protecting access to shells and the environment.

When I wear my shell necklace, I'm wearing an ancient practice around my neck, imbued with stories of women's lives, Country and kinship. I am wearing lowanna tunapry (women's knowledge).[10, 11] Tasmanian Aboriginal women have always made shell necklaces. It is a practice that has endured, and evolved, through Tasmania's ruinous Black War and postcolonial years. Gathering women painstakingly collect, prepare and string the shells. The maireener shells were collected in the shallow coastal waters, where they were pulled from the seaweed to which they were usually attached. The shells were then threaded on kangaroo-tail sinews or on string made from natural fibres and smoked over a fire. Then by rubbing the shells in the grass, the outer coating was removed to reveal the pearly surface beneath. They were later polished with penguin or muttonbird oil.

Aunty Patsy Cameron, also a Pairrebeenne/Trawlwoolway shell stringer born on Flinders Island, explains that the women pierced each shell with a tool made from the eye tooth of a kangaroo that is embedded in the jawbone.[12] While some of the processes for preparing the shells have changed over time, the value and utility of Aboriginal women's kinship is evident in the sustained shell-stringing practice against the backdrop of cultural loss that colonialism brought to Trouwerner. When clanswomen gather to string their shells, they know the history of the shells and they read the coastal seasons, and the weather and tide patterns that enable them to know when it is the right time to collect the shells. Coming together and sharing knowledge, as they have done for thousands of years, strengthens the women's kinship, Law and roles.

The way in which women are connected to place deeply influences their ways of knowing, their notions of wisdom and morality, and conventions of gender. The concept of 'relationality' is central to the kinship and connectedness women have with one another and the knowledge systems they are responsible for. Engaging actively with Country and Mother Earth is a foundation of this kinship. When women gather, they are listening to and learning from Country, and it in turn provides the knowledge needed to sustain their lives. So as the clanswomen of Trouwerner gather to collect shells, they also gather intimate knowledge of Country. The knowledge, which in this case is held by women, then serves to provide for all. Other examples of women's kinship can be seen in stories of birthing, child rearing and the keeping of sacred or secret knowledge that maintain women's connection to place and Country.

When my daughters sit at Little Musselroe Bay, learning their culture and connecting to the place where once their matriarchal ancestors would hunt, sing and care for their children, they too are connected through place and relationships. But there are significant pieces of the puzzle missing for them – language, for example. As a cultural practice that has been particularly targeted in genocidal policies worldwide, language is a primary holder of cultural identity. Due to colonialism's strategy of dismantling Aboriginal cultural infrastructure, language loss is a common experience across Australia.

Languages are living entities that connect people to Country, culture and ancestors. They offer a frame within which meaning is made of the world and provide the tools for conveying thoughts, ideas, concepts and feelings. Languages develop in the context of social and cultural values. Some Aboriginal languages, for example, do not contain the concept of ownership but rather construct meaning and understanding of the world according to relational values. The word for 'moon' might depend on who the speaker is, taking into account their gender, eldership, knowledge, etc. Elders and specialists in language revival speak of language as health, as the foundation for strong cultural identity and wellbeing. They see the process of language retrieval itself as a healing process that strengthens spirit and connects people deeply to their Country and their ancestors. The connectedness between language and health is the same as the connectedness between Country and health: there is balance and symbiotic relationship and the state of one affects the other.

The words on the back of Aunty Joy's book *Welcome to Country* are: 'Wominjeka Wurundjeri balluk yearmenn koondee bik',[13] a welcome to the lands of the Wurundjeri in Woiwurrung language. Living on Wurundjeri Country, I hear these words spoken a lot. The sentiment of the words is generosity, but their sound when spoken always makes me feel I am hearing the breath of the ancestors. The critical status of Indigenous languages globally was recognised by the United Nations for the International Decade of Indigenous Languages 2022–2032. In 1788, over 250 Indigenous languages were spoken across the Australian continent, with approximately 800 varieties. In 2016, there were 120 languages remaining and in 2019, 90 per cent were considered endangered.[14] Early colonial practices sought to eradicate Aboriginal languages and subsequent social and political pressures meant they remained dormant. As a result, over 80 per cent of Aboriginal people today speak Aboriginal English, a variety of Standard English that has enabled Aboriginal people to adapt to policies that forbade the use of traditional language.[15] Kriol is another type of hybrid Aboriginal language that developed; it draws on both traditional language and Standard Australian English.[16] Languages are part of our human heritage and their protection for future generations is vital. They are precious and a resource for supporting health and maintaining cultural continuity. We have much to learn from them.

Country, kinship, language, religion and economy integrate human and spiritual worlds, support wellness and are upheld by ritual and practices that sustain life. My own Country holds a celestial blueprint for living and navigating the landscapes. As Aunty Patsy Cameron has described,[17] the clanspeople of northeastern Trouwerner used the night sky and age-old astronomical knowledge to safely navigate the coastal environment on which their livelihood was centred. Reading the stars across the sky guided everyday practice such as hunting, harvesting of foods including swan and yolla eggs, and the collection of seasonal foods. Sky knowledge provided information about seasonal shifts, weather patterns and the ocean's currents, all important for ensuring food production. But it was not only the ability to read the stars that was important. How the clanspeople of the Coastal Plains Nation understood their lives and its meaning was also held in the celestial world.

In the oral traditions of Aboriginal peoples, scientific knowledge is embedded within religion and the Dreaming, and is held and protected in knowledge archives, passed from generation to generation. For the people of Trouwerner, Sky Country held within its stories the lives of Ancestral Spirits. In his journal, George Augustus Robinson records in August 1831 the Coastal Plains creation story that Mannalargenna told him, a story of how humans and fire came to earth from the sky. The story is only briefly recorded, with many inconsistencies. When Robinson asked him who made the black man [sic], Mannalargenna said that it was two Ancestral Sky Beings in the Milky Way who made humans, rivers and fire; their names were Pumpermehowlle and Pineterrinner.[18] The Ancestral Beings are said to be men who use the Milky Way as their road and have Mars as their foot. Astronomical studies suggest that the sky spirits are Castor and Pollux, the two brightest stars in the Gemini constellation. During the month of May, just after nightfall, Mars is positioned northwest on the horizon, at the feet of the Gemini twins, who use the Milky Way as their road, just before they disappear below the horizon at sunset, as described by Mannalargenna.[19] While incomplete and fractured, this Dreaming story would once have governed significant portions of life for the

Coastal Plains Nation of Trouwerner. Our challenge now is to work toward rebuilding our stories so they can be passed to future generations; as we rebuild these, so too do we rebuild our identities, our sense of place and therefore our health.

Health is also intimately connected to our economy. How an economy considers health and the conditions that affect it says a lot about what we value as a society – the large and persistent gap in expenditure on health care for Aboriginal and Torres Strait Islander people, for example, or the slow and long-overdue expenditure on climate action. The structure of the economy itself, however, is of more concern when understanding how Aboriginal health and wellness have economic value. Traditional Aboriginal economies have a depth far greater than the notion of a subsistence economy suggests. Land holds a central place, with cultural, social and spiritual practices enabling a robust economy that is crucial for good health.

Country and Law are key features of an Aboriginal economic system; kinship and totemic structures, for example, ensured resources were distributed sustainably and equitably. The economic environment within which Aboriginal people live and participate has changed fundamentally since colonisation. The dominant Western economic model is based on a theory of human capital that privileges monetary wealth. Dispossession of ancestral lands and cultural decimation have left Aboriginal people and economies in a void; no longer able to effectively engage in a traditional economy,

Aboriginal people are also left at the margins of the mainstream Australian economy. Within these margins, engagement in the economy is often through a deficit means that ascribes failure or lack of achievement, such as chronic welfare dependence or conditions of program funding that only account for low improvement rather than thriving successes. Aboriginal people are motivated by their sense of belonging, identity, community and connection to Country and culture,[20] but their economic engagement has diminished from that of prospering to that of survival, and health and wellness have suffered as a result.

Uncle Bruce Pascoe in his book *Dark Emu* describes many of the industries of the pre-contact Aboriginal economy. Agriculture, aquaculture, engineering and manufacturing, among others, are fundamental in Uncle Bruce's work toward building an understanding of the economic and socio-political sophistication of traditional Aboriginal life. A particular point he makes in the book is about the relationship between the economy and the spiritual world. Conveying a story about the relationship between killer whales and the people of the Yuin Nation, Uncle Bruce describes a 'ritualised interaction'.[21] A fire ceremony on the land would initiate the herding of large whales by killer whales to the bay, enabling them to be harvested by the people. The sharing economy would benefit the Yuin people and their neighbouring clans but also, importantly, the killer whales themselves, who were rewarded with the harvested large whales' tongues. This practice offered greater reward than food. The interaction with the killer whales rested on a long relationship with their ancestors, as 'the Yuin believe that after death they return as killer whales'.[22] The practice offered social, cultural and spiritual engagement that forms the basis of an Aboriginal economy and therefore health.

The connection between economic necessities and spiritual or cultural practices can be seen in the traditional Aboriginal economy across the country. Wil-im-ee Moor-ring,[23] for example, is a greenstone quarry in central Victoria on the lands of the Wurundjeri people and close to Taungurung and Dja Dja Wurrung lands. The quarry is heritage listed and is under the care of the Wurundjeri Woi Wurrung Cultural Heritage Aboriginal Corporation. A ngurungaeta of the Wurundjeri Wilam, Billibellary played a central role in the management and maintenance of the quarry. He was born in 1799 and was a signatory to the Batman Treaty in 1835 on the banks of the Birrarung (Yarra River). But it was his Elder, Ningulabul, a revered songmaker, who had old authority and proprietorial rights over the quarry. These stories have been generously shared with me over the years and have contributed to the teaching and learning of many students who study on Wurundjeri Country.

Wil-im-ee Moor-ring is known to have been the principal source of axe stone across southeastern Australia. Social and sacred or religious relations underpinned the quarry's production of stone and its trade. Many groups travelled great distances to negotiate the exchange of items for the greenstone of the quarry.[24] It was highly sought after and would feature in large trade gatherings for which spears and possum skin cloaks would be traded.[25] In distinct non-random distribution patterns, hatchet heads made from the stone have been found up to 1000 kilometres from the quarry, in areas where other stone of equal utility was also quarried. The greenstone sourced from Wil-im-ee Moor-ring is said to have had far greater importance than the utilitarian benefits of trade and was prized for its cosmological and ceremonial symbolism.[26]

Such an economy ensured good relations with people further afield and with the spiritual world; such relationships helped people to live healthy lives on Country.

Aboriginal people wish to engage in the dominant economy to ensure a quality of life, and good health, that is commensurate with what they had prior to their dispossession. The messages from Elders, communities and the research that is being done in this area are clear – our culture has the answers to our health. Revitalising our culture and its practices is vital to ensuring the continuity of the oldest living culture in the world. The important part is providing the right conditions to enable our cultures to thrive.

8

ABORIGINAL WORLDVIEWS IN MAINSTREAM SERVICES

FIONA STANLEY

I am a non-Aboriginal woman trained in Western medicine and public health; I have worked closely with Aboriginal researchers for over forty years. I have talked and listened to them, read their papers and others they have recommended, visited communities and gone out on Country with Elders. Over this time, I have observed the dramatic rebirth of Aboriginal knowledge, and how these researchers are using this knowledge to improve the health and wellbeing of First Nations populations. The amazing survival and revitalisation of Aboriginal worldviews and ways of doing is more than admirable; it is astonishing. This trend is taking place after more than 200 years of attempts to eradicate it. What is even more remarkable is that many of the Elders still hold significant knowledge.

Wongi Elder Geoffrey Stokes arranged an extraordinary session for me and Telethon Kids Institute staff out on his Country. Two of his colleagues had prepared a two-hour presentation on traditional foods and medicines, with a long trestle table displaying leaves, oils, gum, fruits, bark and food derived from the land. All the staff were astounded to discover the breadth and depth of this knowledge. I asked Geoff and his colleagues if they were 'specialists' in this knowledge; 'No,' they said, 'we were all taught this from our parents and grandparents.'

Aboriginal scholars have also been able to tap back into material held in places such as AIATSIS, libraries, museums and other collections. I recall a marvellous example when the stories of famous Kimberley artist Queenie McKenzie were recorded by Dr Pat Vinnicombe, an anthropologist and rock art expert. After Queenie died, the tapes were given to the women Elders in the Warmun community. Once the women had heard the tapes and realised that they described the ways of their ancestors, they worked together to bring back the knowledges to the children and young people in the Warmun community. They told me that they were able to bring back some of the lore, songs and ways that had been lost. Shirley Purdie, former Chair of the Warmun community, gave me a beautiful book of Queenie's paintings, side by side with photos of Country. The knowledge was passed on again through story and paintings.

Michael Woodley and Lorraine Coppin lead the Juluwarlu Aboriginal Corporation in Roebourne, in the Pilbara, Western

Australia. They invited some Yindjibarndi Elders to visit Juluwarlu and share some of their deep knowledge of traditional ways, which the Elders had learned by being brought up on Country. When Michael and Lorraine showed them Google maps of the Country belonging to the Yindjibarndi, the Elders excitedly named, in language, all the trees, rocks and sites of cultural and spiritual significance and told their histories. They were also able to identify birthing trees and botanical species used in ceremony. When shown photos of the native animals, the Elders named them in language and recalled the stories about these animals and how they were hunted and used. Two beautiful books have been published by Juluwarlu and these and the stories are being passed on to future generations.[1]

HOW CULTURE AND TRADITIONAL KNOWLEDGES CAN BE USED TO PROVIDE EFFECTIVE HEALTH CARE

Aboriginal health researchers know how culture and traditional knowledges can be used to change services from Western paradigms to provide the safest and most effective ways of care. Due to the dramatic changes in diseases brought on by dispossession and marginalisation (obesity, diabetes, heart disease, substance abuse, STDs, rheumatic heart disease, mental-health problems), these researchers also realise that partnering with Western knowledge is essential. My role and that of other non-Indigenous allies is to encourage and enable this to happen by any means that we have. While the power comes when these Western medical practices are imbedded in Aboriginal worldviews, such as within Aboriginal community-controlled organisations, the examples presented in this chapter describe how Aboriginal worldviews can be incorporated into mainstream health services.

The first well-documented model is led by Dr Michael Wright, a Noongar researcher from Western Australia. Michael is one of the scholars with whom I work. The project is called '*Debakarn Koorliny Wangkiny*: steady walking and talking using First Nations-led participatory action research methodologies to build relationships'.[2] This paper starts with a quote from an Elder: 'See us as your cultural carpenters: we'll help shape you for this work. By the end you won't know yourselves.'[3]

The method Michael and his research colleagues taught us is called Aboriginal Community Participation Action Research, and it was used over the years of this project. It is a complete reversal of how non-Indigenous health and medical research is done. In mainstream research, the academic researchers decide on the ideas and hypotheses without any contact or input from the community. The ideas come from the literature (dominated by non-Indigenous scientific methods) and the information (data) being sought is decided by the chief investigator and their team of non-Indigenous researchers. When the data is collected and computerised, the analysis is done without any input or consent from the people from whom it was obtained, and the papers, books and talks are written without their knowledge or interpretation.

In Aboriginal Community Participation Action Research, the community is engaged from the beginning to the end of the process: the idea of the research questions, how they are asked, who should be selected, what data is to be collected and how the data is computerised are all done in close collaboration and in a trusting partnership. As well, the important analysis and interpretation are done with a full understanding of how the findings relate to the Indigenous circumstance.

The *Looking Forward* Project aimed to decolonise the management of First Nations people with serious mental illness in an area of suburban Perth that had high rates of suicide and self-harm, alcohol and drug use, and psychosis. Michael Wright's PhD investigated the reasons why most Aboriginal people in these suburbs did not use mainstream services, despite being at high risk of serious mental illness and having high needs.

The underlying thinking was that if colonisation led to dispossession of land, history and culture, then decolonising is reconnecting to land, history and culture. There was a dual focus, which aimed to incorporate local Indigenous knowledge into the research process and to use the research to mitigate the damaging effects of ignoring Aboriginal worldviews. The approach was to ask the local Elders, as the holders of Noongar knowledges, to talk to the service providers about their lived experience.

Twenty-two Elders, ten partner organisations, three peak agencies, one large hospital, four mainstream NGO mental-health providers and two alcohol and drug support services engaged in the project, which has now been running for some years.

The Elders told their detailed stories of how colonisation had affected them, their families and communities; how it had taken away all those aspects of their world that were necessary for good lives and healthy living. The service providers heard these stories, often feeling awkward and unsure, but coming to a realisation of how important listening to the stories was, to understand the patterns of illness they were seeing. The stories clearly explained why the previous services' frameworks had failed Aboriginal people so profoundly.

An important aspect of this was that 'elders [were] talking to elders'.[4] That is, the service providers whom the Noongar Elders were talking to were those in charge of the services – CEOs, heads of departments, leaders of community services, etc. This transfer of knowledge was based on meaningful, purposeful and honest relationships, which was key to its success. As an advocate and mentor of this work, I remember the faces of the Elders as they planned how the project would work and how excited and enthusiastic they were to be taking on these important roles. There were major shifts in understanding the impact of their history by the mainstream services. The service providers realised that they needed to offer a more family-based service that did not focus only on the person with mental illness in a hospital clinic or service office. They realised that family relationships were crucial both to understanding the underlying psychiatric problem and more importantly how it should be managed. These were crucial changes to services, particularly in the commitment to employing Aboriginal staff. This process was extremely challenging in the Westernised contexts, where there had been such an imbalance, and the dominant culture had complete control over knowledge, practice and cultural environments.

During the meeting, one of the Elders said, 'You know all about us but we don't know nothing about yous.'[5] This was a pivotal moment – suddenly the service providers could see that a two-way exchange was necessary and would make a positive impact. Sharing personal stories is not a normal part of professional spaces, despite mainstream mental-health workers demanding all the intimate details of their patients. At last, service providers were also able to tell their stories – the two-way storytelling was truth-telling. And this truth-telling became part of the shared goal for human rights and systematic change, to remove racism from the services and make them welcoming. 'I feel safe, I can cry here,' as one of the Elders said, was a measure of a relationship not a service.

Collectively the team listed several conditions that enhanced the success of working together towards a Noongar worldview. They were: 'Being motivated, being committed, being present, being teachable, staying connected, respecting status and continually weaving.'[6] The research team and all the participants observed that Noongar culture prospered and adapted to the new and developing mainstream framework, which of course was also adapting and responding to the knowledge of the Elders. The racist stereotypes of Aboriginal people, as useless and helpless victims, not following orders nor responding to Western medical environments, slowly morphed into a view that was more understanding of land, culture, relationships and mental health in the Noongar people.

The *Looking Forward* Project has been a success and is now being implemented across the metropolitan area of Perth. The team is evaluating the impact of the changes and specifically asking: 'What would a service that is culturally safe for Aboriginal people look like? What should we measure to see a change in the service? How do we measure these changes?'[7]

The Elders and researchers described three areas to measure what success looked like. The first was relationships between those using and providing the services; the second was the level of employment and capacity building of an Aboriginal workforce; and third was whether Aboriginal people felt culturally safe, welcome and secure. Involving family and caregivers and focusing on a strengths-based approach, not on deficits, were more important than improving mental health.

These processes really challenged Western medical service thinking, funding and accountability. They clearly made the case for how to change services so they are acceptable to First Nations people, are trusted and used by them. They have completely changed the relationships between the mainstream service providers and the First Nations people with serious mental illness, and their families. The most important 'take home message' here is that Elders were acknowledged (and paid) as co-researchers; that the focus on strengths more than deficits was crucial; that the role of family and community was acknowledged and encouraged; and that many of the 'measures' that they valued were unable to be measured by Western methods. This included the feelings of Elders and the trust of the people using the services. Maybe there are lessons here for our Western mental-health services too? And can these methods be used in other mainstream services that are failing Aboriginal families?

Ngullak Koolunga Ngullak Koort (Our children our heart) is a research project at the Telethon Kids Institute in Western Australia run by a group of Noongar Elders – Millie Penny and Charmaine Pell – and facilitated and led by Ngunnawal postdoctoral researcher Sharynne Hamilton. The group of Elders wanted their knowledge, wisdom and expertise to be adopted so that the high rates of child removals and inappropriate out-of-home care in Western Australia could be reduced. The Elders developed child protection principles and practice recommendations. They have called for a recognition of the intergenerational harm caused by the Stolen Generation policies from 1901 to 1975, as recorded in the *Bringing Them Home* Report[8] in 1997, and they want this used as a foundation for formulating future policies and practices.

This applied research uses the same Aboriginal Community Participation Action Research methods described earlier, capturing all the wisdom of the grandparents and parents, and asking them for their stories of how they were treated by these government services. The Elders described how their families experienced these child protection and family services in the past and how little has really changed. They spoke of their intense distrust of 'the welfare', which continues to flow through all Aboriginal communities in Western Australia. They called for child protection services to harness resources and connections from the vast social networks that exist in Aboriginal communities, being respectful of families, building trust and relationships and finding community-led, local solutions for children at risk. They suggested using Aboriginal family-led decision-making forums that prioritised 'our voices'. Some families are scared to access any welfare services, fearing that they will be reported, or their children removed, as they and their parents may have been. As Ngunnawal woman, Dr Sharynne Hamilton said, 'Children miss out on health checks or schooling: Historical trauma and distrust run very deep in our community.'[9]

This critically important work recognises that:

> the Nanas are the social and community glue that keep our families and communities together. The Elders continually raise the concern that the work of the Nanas is unnoticed and unsupported. In our communities all our sisters are aunties, all our nans are mums, all our brothers are uncles, all our pops are dads. All our kids are cousins. We need a much greater understanding among non-Aboriginal people about cultural differences in what it means to be part of an Aboriginal kinship network and what this can provide to bolster the safety of children to live with kin, in their communities and embedded in their culture and language.[10]

If those running the mainstream child protection, health and other welfare services appreciated that this network exists throughout all Western Australian communities, not only could they provide better care for children, but they would also save significant child protection expenses. They would not fail Aboriginal children and families; they would reduce the numbers of Aboriginal youth failing in school and being detained by the justice system. The Elders say, 'this should be one of our biggest investments'. 'What we have done in our work is to combine our two knowledge systems together. We brought together the cultural wisdom and knowledge of the Elders and the community with the academic knowledge of regulatory theory.'[11] Regulatory pyramid models[12] consider the families' cultures, behaviours, circumstances and environments; they hold the community at the centre and aim for cooperation and self-regulation.[13]

Mainstream services all too frequently remove a child first and ask questions later, and as the reasons given for removing 84 per cent of children are unsubstantiated,[14] this means that many suffer unwarranted trauma (again and again).

> If saying 'sorry' meant anything – asking questions about historical involvement of the state and hearing these stories of our families should invite a fundamentally different response to the family. A unique and individual response, led by our Elders, led by Aboriginal Community organisations and the community to redress the harms that a family could have suffered over many generations. Responses where the focus is on recovery, on providing recovery pathways, and on ensuring everything is provided to safely care for children with their families, in their communities and on their country. These changes would turn hollow words to healing.[15]

Western European knowledges are, and were, based on very different cultural thinking from those of First Nations people; the European system suggested a hierarchy of perfection, with plants and minerals at the bottom and European humans at the top. This hierarchical view of life extended to the racial, which positioned some humans, such as they themselves, at the top, in the belief that they were more culturally advanced and hence were given the power to dominate all other worldviews. European nations did this by colonising many Indigenous communities around the world, in ignorance of the extraordinarily rich cultures that their invasive colonisation destroyed, diminished and tried to eradicate.

I recall going out on Noongar Ballardong Yuet Country with my close friend and esteemed Elder Dr Noel Nannup. He has a profound knowledge of Country, its beginnings, its plants and animals, and how First Nations beliefs worked harmoniously for a good life. The importance of relationships between kin and between kin groups and their Country was beautiful to hear. Another of the group, a non-Aboriginal woman, asked Noel, 'Why don't you hate us, why aren't you angry?'

Noel, who is the gentlest of people, replied, 'Where would that get me? I will let the spirits manage that. But if I can tell you about my Country and its beauty, then you may appreciate how much we have suffered because we have lost so much of it.'

IMPACT OF COLONISATION ON HEALTH AND WELLBEING

Colonisation was a brutal process that eroded cultural knowledge and practices, along with language, and caused the separation of families and loss of access to land. Figure 1 shows the impact of these changes on the pathways into the health and social issues affecting many First Nations people today. All Indigenous groups with this history suffer the same problems as our Aboriginal people.

Impact of white colonisation on Aboriginal health today

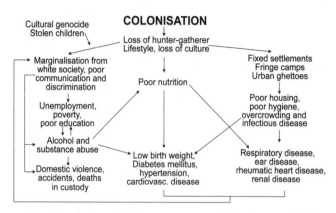

FIGURE 1: This diagram shows the disastrous impact of colonisation on Aboriginal populations in Australia to explain their current circumstances and why there is a 'gap' compared to non-Aboriginal outcomes.[16]

These are not Aboriginal problems; non-Indigenous people would have had these problems too if we had had this history.

Health and other services that affect health, such as birthing, education, housing, child protection and justice, have been developed by the mainstream Western culture in ignorance of First Nations knowledges. Ignoring Aboriginal worldviews and knowledges in this way is symptomatic of the various forms of racism, at times extreme, that exist in virtually all non-Indigenous controlled services, and it has an impact on every aspect of Aboriginal people's lives. These siloed Western services do not manage Aboriginal health (or other) issues well and they can do more harm than good in reducing the gap between Aboriginal and Torres Strait Islanders and non-Indigenous Australians.

There are two main reasons why successive governments have failed to close the gap; one is that they defunded, or underfunded, effective Aboriginal-controlled services, and secondly, they implemented expensive but ineffective mainstream services. The federal, state and territory government bureaucrats may have good intentions towards improving Aboriginal health and wellbeing, but these services usually fail because they ignore the Indigenous worldview, they make Aboriginal people feel ashamed and unwelcome – put simply, they are racist. They fail because they are developed without an understanding of the root causes of the problems, often with dire consequences for First Nations people. These services fail because of Aboriginal people's lack of trust in them.

In the early 2000s, the Secretariat for National Aboriginal and Islander Child Care (SNAICC) with support from the federal government, supported over seventy Aboriginal community-controlled child and family centres all around the country. One of the most well-known is the Child and Parent Centre in the Fitzroy Valley, Western Australia, set up by senior Bunuba woman June Oscar (now national Social Justice Commissioner) and Emily and Maureen Carter. They manage this service from the Marninwarntikura Women's Resource Centre. Marninwarntikura is a Walmajarri word meaning 'women belonging together'. The centre provides trauma healing and support for the early years and also runs a major program to manage and prevent Fetal Alcohol Syndrome. As well, women and others work in social enterprises, there is an art studio, a women's shelter, domestic violence prevention and a legal unit, which are all run by the Marninwarntikura Women's Resource Centre.

These Aboriginal-led services were not only in remote areas of the nation, but also in rural and urban areas (another well-known centre is Bubup Wilam in metropolitan Melbourne, run by Lisa Thorpe), and they partnered with government departments such as Education and Health. The centres were much more effective than any government services run for Aboriginal families in Australia. Their results included achieving closing-the-gap targets such as more children being healthy and ready for school and increasing Year 12 completion rates.

In 2015, in spite of these services being shown to be effective, they were defunded by the Coalition Government, which suggested that they be funded by state and territory governments. Instead of supporting these services, the new federal childcare funding was aimed at getting (non-Indigenous) women back to work after having a child. Childcare subsidies to access private childcare services were given to women if they were working or training, thus excluding many Aboriginal families.

Despite protests and lobbying for the Aboriginal services to continue, since being defunded many services have struggled to keep working effectively. The result has been an increase in child and youth problems nationally – health, mental health, educational and crime – with politicians and the community asking why so many Aboriginal kids are 'going off the rails'. The cost to the community and the taxpayer of this action is huge and it is anguishing for Aboriginal organisations to see their families and young people suffering.

If programs are developed in complete isolation from the local culture and remotely from community, they tend to cause further dislocation and loss of self-esteem. A well-known, expensive, punitive and traumatising mainstream service was the 2007 Northern Territory Emergency Response, also known as The Intervention. Done without any Aboriginal consultation, the defence forces and white bureaucrats went in with very restrictive practices, and many aspects of The Intervention were humiliating and went against human rights. The appalling effect was an *increase* in child sexual abuse in the Northern Territory every year after that intervention.[17] This 'service' was the federal government's response to the *Little Children are Sacred* Report, which contained recommendations from Aboriginal families and leaders that were completely ignored. How would you feel if this was your family, your place, your child?

The inclusion of cultural values, such as acknowledging family relationships and kinship groups, engaging with Elders who hold the intergenerational knowledge, and involving the whole family in providing care for children, would mean that Aboriginal communities can set their own parameters for restoring sustainable relationships that allow services to work for them. A major factor here is *trust*. Many years ago, I sent one of my Master of Public Health students to Kalgoorlie to ask a large sample of Aboriginal people why they did not use mainstream services.[18] The answers were disturbing to read: how Aboriginal women were made to feel they were 'bad mothers', were 'dirty and smelly' and ignorant of how to look after or treat their children. Also, there were too many stories of children not getting proper treatment when the mothers did take them to the service; some of these children died because the mainstream service providers did not give appropriate care. There is a saying among white service providers: 'Give them Panadol and send them home.' This occurs too frequently with serious diseases such as rheumatic heart disease, with children and adults not being followed up for their penicillin treatment and thus developing heart complications that are fatal.[19]

Aboriginal leadership and employing Aboriginal people restore trust and deliver services that understand current Aboriginal circumstances and fears. They also increase the self-esteem of those employed and those who are served.

The case for change in Aboriginal services is clear, with the gaps in targets for health and wellbeing showing little or no improvement and in some cases widening. Some of these are because non-Indigenous rates are improving faster than the Indigenous ones, but many are showing worsening trends, as demonstrated in the *Closing the Gap* Report of 2023.[20] It is obvious that the ways of working with and delivering health and other services to First Nations people need to change dramatically.

One of the learnings is to acknowledge that Aboriginal culture is dynamic and adapting. It is not an archaic, interesting ancient but dead culture to be read about in *National Geographic* magazines! Aboriginal knowledges can be adapted to bring new ways of interacting and relating into mainstream services for health and wellbeing, and not just for Aboriginal people. Using these methods, as in the projects described above, many of the mainstream providers and staff began to see that these new ways of working together were better for everyone.

I wonder if there would be some way of insisting on this cultural transmission of services for Aboriginal people. One way would be to accredit those services that have the characteristics that Aboriginal consultants identify as crucial. If they have met these guidelines, they can be funded to provide services, and if they do not, then their funding is withdrawn. Usually it is the funding of the Aboriginal-controlled services that is withdrawn.

The Voice to Parliament would have been the perfect vehicle to encourage these approaches. During the campaign, I wrote with my Aboriginal colleagues to make the case for how a Voice would make such a difference to improving health for Indigenous people.[21,22] We now wonder how hard it is going to be to change our mainstream services so that the Aboriginal people who use them feel that they are being cared for. I believe that these are great models of Aboriginal knowledges for changing ineffective, expensive and damaging services into effective ones. If this can be done, albeit over a lengthy period, then can it be used in other service settings? What can we learn from Aboriginal Community Participation Action Research to apply to the racist, unwelcoming, culturally insecure services that have too often become the norm?

9

AN INDIGENOUS-LED HEALTH RESEARCH AGENDA

SANDRA EADES AND FIONA STANLEY

Imagine being invited to take part in a research project that will look at ear disease in your children. A group of powerful non-Indigenous doctors have decided that they want to find out why so many Aboriginal children have serious ear disease. You are a mum of three children, all of whom have had such bad ears that it is interfering with their ability to hear, and they are having trouble at school. You receive a letter from these researchers who work in the capital city, a long way from the regional town where you live. They are hoping that you will agree to take part in a survey – they are asking you to fill in a questionnaire and to agree to have your children examined by an ear-health doctor. They promise that if any problems are found, your children will receive free ear health care, including surgery should the children need it.

You give permission and answer the questionnaire and your children are examined. Some months later you read an article in the local newspaper – or worse, watch a television program – reporting that children in families living in your town, in poor circumstances, and who have limited access to ear health services, have high rates of ear disease and hearing loss. The paper quotes the doctors as saying that the main reasons for the high rates of disease are poverty, inadequate and overcrowded housing, and families who are ignorant about the disease and how to get help for their children. The image this creates in the report and among your community is that you and others like you are the cause of the problem. There is no explanation of your lived experience or your understanding of why your children have ear disease.

The project does not result in any improvement in housing or financial circumstances, nor does it help you to get appropriate care more quickly. This is an appalling result from research that, in a grant application, promised that the information obtained would guide improved outcomes for Aboriginal children with ear disease.

Could this have been done differently, so the doctors engaged fully with families in that community, to ascertain what their issues were in relation to their children's health, and how best to help the children be healthy? And how different might it have been if the person running the whole study was an Aboriginal doctor or nurse who understood the Indigenous worldviews that you had about your own circumstances?

In recent times, Aboriginal researchers in Australia have managed to influence the funding of research. They have also started to influence how data is managed to enable communities to have control over data relating to them, through data sovereignty, and to shape research through the input of Indigenous voices, opinions and worldviews.

At a recent round table, some Elders said to me (Fiona), 'Is this research really necessary? We know what to do.' And, 'Are they doing research for research's sake and not for us?'

The major challenge with any medical (and social) investigations is that we know that the solutions are to intervene early in the disease process rather than waiting until the damage is done. In relation to Indigenous people, virtually all their poor health and social circumstances stem from the adverse impacts of colonisation – due to poverty, marginalisation and racism, as explored in other chapters of this book. The way studies are done has improved more recently, mostly because they are led by Aboriginal researchers, and more research is done in collaboration, involving community participation. However, there is still this glaringly obvious situation where the solution to improving health hardly needs any more investigation – it needs action to implement basic changes to improve living conditions, and to overcome poverty, racism and exclusion.

Aboriginal people have rightly been critical of the research that has been carried out over the last two centuries, particularly that done by anthropologists and social and medical researchers. Many of these non-Indigenous academics and researchers built their careers around intensive and sometimes invasive studies of First Nations people, with no inclusion, understanding or benefit to Aboriginal people.[1] In fact, much of it did harm by describing Aboriginal people in negative ways; they were angry that these studies were done on them but not with them.[2] These studies produced many PhDs and led to fame for white researchers, but left out Aboriginal people, and the studies certainly were not used in ways that were beneficial. Despite this, a number of Aboriginal people could see that research was a good tool for advocacy and elevating Aboriginal voices. Not surprisingly, though, they were questioned about why they wanted to be involved in such projects. The feeling in the 1980s and 1990s was that Aboriginal people were the most researched people in the country, with no clear benefit to people or communities.

NHMRC ROADMAPS

What happens in Australia now? How is health and medical research conducted? Who influences which projects are funded? And how are these projects assessed before the money is wasted on studies that may never help the people that they are investigating?

Australia set up the major funding agency for health and medical research in 1937, the National Health and Medical Research Council (NHMRC), and until the 1990s it was dominated by white (mostly male) researchers and experts who decided the areas of research and who would get funded. Aboriginal and Torres Strait Islander health and medical research was led by non-Indigenous researchers, few of whom had any understanding of the First Nations knowledges influencing health, nor any real conception of the positive power of culture. Few employed Aboriginal people in their investigations, nor were Aboriginal people consulted as to how information was used. Most non-Indigenous researchers had a reasonable idea of the adverse effects of colonisation and the Stolen Generations, and paper after paper chronicled the appalling state of Aboriginal health.[3]

As non-Indigenous researchers and public health professionals we (Fiona) did not want to damage the image of Aboriginal people. Our aim was to get our governments, service providers and the media to push for change to improve the health and wellbeing of Aboriginal and Torres Strait Islander people. While it did result in more interest, it also made many Aboriginal people feel shame and hopelessness about their situation. We know that these circumstances can all be explained by the negative impacts on the lives of Aboriginal people since colonisation. And it did little to raise the image of Aboriginal people in the general population. Sadly, the media and many non-Indigenous people in Australia still have this negative image of people living in squalid circumstances with chronic disease and substance abuse. It makes us frustrated that the media will show footage of families in squalor rather than the ten new First Nations doctors and nurses graduating from universities.

STRENGTHS-BASED APPROACH TO ABORIGINAL HEALTH RESEARCH

Fiona, as an institute director and leading Australian researcher, and I (Sandra), as a budding Aboriginal health researcher, were involved in exploring epidemiological descriptions of the gap, looking at the deficit model. While there are still Aboriginal people today with health and other problems, they are not universal, and it is always beneficial to look at both sides of the story. Papers and media articles describe, for example, 'low rates' of Year 12 retention, but nearly 60 per cent of Aboriginal kids completed Year 12 in 2021 (for non-Aboriginal youth it was 79 per cent).[4] We need to acknowledge those 60 per cent who, in spite of being at risk, have done so well. Fiona and I were a part of the movement to bring a strengths-based approach to Aboriginal health research as we realised how damaging this negative way of looking at things was. It still held sway during the early years when I was completing my PhD in medicine to become the first Aboriginal doctor to be trained both in medicine and in research in Australia. My PhD study, which Fiona supervised, was entitled 'Bibbulung Gnarneep' or 'Solid Kid' in Noongar.[5] I wanted to look at what kept Noongar babies healthy and solid in the first year of life, rather than just looking at what led to poor health.

When I started working as a general practitioner at the Perth Aboriginal Medical Service (now Derbarl Yerrigan Health Service), I was struck by how the PAMS, serving Aboriginal people with great health needs, had very little access to evidence-based medicine and research that was so widespread in the tertiary university hospitals where I had trained in medicine. My interest in research stemmed from my belief that research was urgently needed to advocate for Aboriginal people's health needs and policy and health service responses. I also realised how important it was for me to succeed as a role model for others coming along in my wake.

In the late 1990s, as more Aboriginal health researchers were trained, NHMRC put these researchers on key committees within the organisation. Hence budding research leaders such as Ian Anderson (the first Aboriginal researcher to receive an NHMRC grant in 1997) and I were invited to serve on Aboriginal advisory committees that influenced the main business of the NHMRC. Little did the organisation know what changes were afoot to improve the culture within it, to enable research that helped rather than damaged First Nations people.

A national government standing committee on Aboriginal health produced a report recommending changes that could help accelerate the pace at which steps were taken to improve the health of Australia's Aboriginal and Torres Strait Islander people.[6] Some of the recommendations of this report were that the NHMRC commit 5 per cent of its budget to focus on Aboriginal and Torres Strait Islander research and particularly to support Aboriginal community-controlled research. I was a member of the NHMRC's strategic Research Agenda Working Group (RAWG) at the time this report was tabled in parliament and the NHMRC was invited to provide a response to this recommendation. Work conducted by RAWG led to national consultation on Aboriginal health research, with the findings informing the development of the first draft 'Roadmap for Aboriginal and Torres Strait Islander Research'.[7]

Real changes in funding for and the support of Aboriginal research within NMHRC came when it adopted the RAWG recommendations in 2002. To date, three rounds of 'roadmaps', which First Nations researchers describe as a set of guidelines developed by Aboriginal people for Aboriginal people, have been published. The first was in 2002, the second in 2010 and the last in

2018, each planning to guide NHMRC investment in First Nations research, to build capacity (more Aboriginal researchers with pathways into research training), and to focus on those research areas that would lead to the greatest improvement in health. Each roadmap developed a ten-year strategic plan to ensure that these aims were met and that they were done in appropriate ways and engaged properly with community members, particularly Elders. The group lobbied for community engagement to be funded from grants and to allow the time to have community engagement in projects.

We often talk about those early days of our work with the NHMRC. I helped lead the first consultation process with John Delaney, who was the Chair of the RAWG committee, and my Aboriginal colleagues Jacinta Elston from James Cook University, Terry Dunbar from the Co-operative Research Centre in Aboriginal and Tropical Health in Darwin, and Aboriginal health leaders Professor Ian Anderson and Professor Shane Houston, and our non-Aboriginal supporters, including Professor Kerin O'Dea. My experience working in research had taught me that we needed Aboriginal people, researchers and policy makers in the same room to discuss what would be needed in a roadmap for Aboriginal health research that drew on Aboriginal perspectives and centred on these in new paths forward. Workshops were held around the country, with Aboriginal researchers, Elders, community leaders and relevant organisations (such as universities and research institutes, state and territory representatives). Fiona recalls attending some of these dialogues with me – it was the first time she had been in a meeting where 75 per cent of those present were First Nations people and non-Indigenous people were in the minority!

Fiona received one of the first major NHMRC grants for training people to develop their skills and capacity in Aboriginal health and medical research. This led to the training of ten outstanding researchers, as she mentioned in her introduction. Through them a range of changes were introduced to ensure that Elders and community members were part of the research team from the beginning. These Community Participation Action Research methods have been described in chapter 7. I, with Fiona and Anne Read (one of our devoted epidemiological researchers who co-supervised me for my PhD), developed the best practice model of having community reference groups for all Indigenous research.[8, 9] Now most Aboriginal research is led by Aboriginal people and some funding organisations will not fund research in Aboriginal health unless the chief investigator is an Indigenous person. What a change for the good!

NO DATA OR RESEARCH ON US WITHOUT US

The most helpful lesson for us, particularly Fiona, was about how interviews to obtain the best data were conducted differently when Aboriginal researchers were in charge. Our Telethon Kids Institute team knew that Aboriginal families were anxious about cot deaths (Sudden Infant Death Syndrome) and they had approached us to help prevent their children from dying. Instead of sending letters inviting them to participate and attaching a two to three-page questionnaire (which was done with non-Indigenous mothers), we personally contacted the mothers and Aboriginal health workers visited them in their homes. They started by 'yarning' to the mums – sharing information as to where they were from, their family and especially about their children. The research questions came after however long it took to develop a trusted relationship with the mother; much more information about her and her mothering was obtained in this caring exchange. Discussions about knowledge of the causes and prevention of cot deaths then followed, with particular reference to how children were cared for in the first year of life.

In some cases, we brought several mothers together with our Elders (Shirley Thorne facilitated this Elders group, some of whom have now passed) on the project, so the mothers felt comfortable about sharing their information. Details about the known risk and protective factors for cot death were shared, such as breast feeding and introduction of solids, smoking, position of baby to sleep and with whom the baby slept. The subsequent analysis and interpretation of the data was done in close consultation with the mothers and Elders. We believe that we had developed the best guidelines for Aboriginal mums because they owned the whole process. Shirley Thorne also led the prevention project, which meant that the mothers and families trusted that information. We realised why preventive health promotion programs often failed Aboriginal people and how we could avoid the waste of ineffective programs developed in isolation from the people they need to serve.

This has been a most important process for me (Fiona) to take part in, as I could see how these methods so clearly worked. In no way did they diminish the integrity of the research. In fact, it was blindingly obvious that such methods were superior to those we used for much of our work. Due to Aboriginal researchers writing up these methods,[10] they are now becoming more widely appreciated and used. I would not conduct any qualitative study with Aboriginal mums now without yarning, nor would I analyse any quantitative data without their input. Otherwise, I would get it wrong, with possibly serious repercussions. 'First do no harm' is in the Hippocratic Oath!

Elders in Western Australia asked the Telethon Kids Institute to run a population survey, as they realised the power of such data. The result was the WA Aboriginal Child Health Survey,[11] which collected information on one in six Aboriginal families all over Western Australia – from urban to remote communities. Aboriginal researchers led the project and many of the interviewers were Indigenous. They visited the communities to collect information on all aspects of these families' lives that influenced their health and social and emotional wellbeing – at home, at school and outside. The most important and unique information was a history of Stolen Generations parents and grandparents being forcibly removed from their families. The Aboriginal Elders and consultants on the survey insisted that we ask these questions. We could never have collected, analysed or interpreted this data without Aboriginal control.

I am still overwhelmed by the fact that we had nearly 90 per cent of Aboriginal families across Western Australia who participated. That is one of the highest response rates we have ever had in any of our studies. I felt immensely proud of this, but it also came with great responsibility, as these families were trusting us with their stories in the hope that the data would improve their lives. Given the low participation rates of many Aboriginal people in research, for care and service attendance, this demonstrated the effects of Aboriginal involvement in the research team. To this day, this survey is the only one in Australia that describes the extent (between 40 and 60 per cent of all families) and the impact (third and fourth generations) of the Stolen Generations on these families.[12]

These early experiences have resulted in research that helps guide state-based and national policies to improve Aboriginal health. Many of the people trained in research by Fiona and others early on are now leading their own research centres and groups to address youth mental-health issues, and novel research based on their own ideas in partnership with communities about how to support Aboriginal young people and families. Throughout Western Australia and nationally, Aboriginal health research is widespread and increasingly led by Aboriginal researchers with genuine partnerships with Aboriginal communities.

The ABC *Four Corners* episode 'Backing Bourke',[13] filmed in 2016, in Bourke, New South Wales, explored what can happen when researchers collect different data from what would be collected in a mainstream research project. The local Aboriginal people shifted the emphasis of data collection from trends in numbers and rates of young offenders to data that described the young person's passage into and through the criminal justice system in Bourke. They also collected additional information about the young people's early life, education, employment, housing, health, child safety, and mental health and substance abuse. The community owned, analysed and used the data to develop the *Maranguka (Helping each other) Program*.[14] This involves the community engaging with a variety of service providers, not just police and the justice system, but also health, education and social services. Informed by data, this community-led justice reinvestment has been implemented in other communities in New South Wales that have high rates of Indigenous incarceration. The Bourke program was presented at an Indigenous Data Sovereignty meeting at the University of Melbourne in 2019, and demonstrated the dramatic reduction in youth contacts with the police and justice system in the town. The young Aboriginal public health research presenter commented that now police had fewer arrests and had more time to spend in recreational activities with Aboriginal youth in the town.

In another example, after a study done by a non-Aboriginal medical student (now doctor) Rosalie Schultz, which showed high rates of infections in pregnancy associated with preterm births and deaths, my (Fiona) research team actively engaged with the Aboriginal families in that region. The answer was clear – Eastern Goldfields Aboriginal families were treated so badly by the mainstream services that they did not use them. This included avoiding mainstream antenatal care, and their babies were at much higher risk. With an enthusiastic group of Aboriginal women, Fiona wrote a grant application to establish a maternal and early childhood program in the Eastern Goldfields, called *Ngunytju Tjitji Pirni – NTP – mothers, grandmothers all together*. It aimed to improve pregnancy and early childhood care and outcomes in Kalgoorlie and surrounding areas. This program was so successful that we had pregnant mums coming in from all over the Goldfields to participate in a service they wanted for their kids. And attendance for antenatal care at twenty weeks rose from less than 20 per cent to more than 80 per cent.

The program's success was achieved through having Aboriginal staff working as 'brokers' to encourage Aboriginal women to use the mainstream services by attending the services with them. Infant vaccination, breast feeding and attendance for ear disease appointments all increased. While I predicted in our grant application that hospitalisations would be reduced, they went up four-fold as the mums trusted the services that were being brokered by the health workers. The women were now being properly treated for their infections in pregnancy. I was still on my learning journey! One of the other results that I had not predicted was the increased levels of self-esteem of the mothers and of the Aboriginal staff. Not only did they love their work but many of them went on to train in health professions. And some of those mothers who had been in the program then came to work in it themselves. NTP was successful because Aboriginal women owned the study and the data, and from this developed how studies should be done. It is another example of Aboriginal control being vastly more successful than mainstream.

INDIGENOUS DATA SOVEREIGNTY

As we discussed above, there are some exciting examples of how radically different outcomes occur when Indigenous communities take control of their own data and how it is used. A major step forward in this respect was the development of Indigenous Data Sovereignty and Indigenous Data Governance.

In Australia in around 2010, major work was done to consult Aboriginal communities about the use of genetic blood samples taken from their members, particularly how it should be used in research or returned to communities. Those consultations occurred with many communities where a priori research over decades resulted in the collection and storage of Aboriginal tissue samples, mostly without consent. At a national and state level, awareness increased about the need for Aboriginal people to be consulted and involved whenever total population data, collected routinely from Aboriginal people by government agencies, was used in research or evaluation projects. No longer could it be taken for granted that such research or reporting about Aboriginal people could be conducted without the involvement of these people in the process.

There is now an exciting and important global Indigenous-led movement to ensure that Aboriginal people hold the right to govern the creation, collection, ownership and application of their data, to 'own' that data; this right has become known as Indigenous Data Sovereignty.[15]

For Indigenous people, data is a cultural, strategic and economic asset, because how it is used can have major positive or negative impacts for them.[16] While Aboriginal people in Australia have always been active in 'data', they have been excluded from the language, control and production of data at community, state and national levels. As discussed earlier, this has often led to suggestions that they were 'the problem', rather than exploring the historical and cultural reasons why people have become unwell. Data collection, management and analysis that takes place within mainstream institutions rarely has any Indigenous input. This in turn often means that the current and future needs of First Nations people are not recognised. For example, the Australian Bureau of Statistics records whether a person is of Aboriginal or Islander descent, but not the language group(s) that describes their original Country and the Country of their ancestors. Many Aboriginal and Torres Strait Islander people we have talked to would like to have national data collected on these because they realise that there is such diversity across different language groups.

In 2018, a meeting of First Nations people from the Australian Indigenous Governance Institute and delegates from the Maiam nayri Wingara Indigenous Data Sovereignty Collective from Aotearoa, was held in Canberra. A national document on data sovereignty, *Indigenous Data Sovereignty Communique*, was produced from this meeting, and delegates endorsed the following statements:

> In Australia, '*Indigenous Data*' refers to information or knowledge, in any format or medium, which is about and may affect Indigenous peoples both collectively and individually.

> '*Indigenous Data Sovereignty*' refers to the right of Indigenous peoples to exercise ownership over Indigenous Data. Ownership of data can be expressed through the creation, collection, access, analysis, interpretation, management, dissemination and reuse of Indigenous Data.

> '*Indigenous Data Governance*' refers to the right of Indigenous peoples to autonomously decide what, how and why Indigenous Data are collected, accessed and used. It ensures that data on or about Indigenous peoples reflects our priorities, values, cultures, worldviews and diversity.[17]

Indigenous Data Sovereignty goes hand in hand with the concept of Aboriginal Community Participation Action Research methods, and with the best practice of employing Community Reference Groups for all Aboriginal research. By following these processes, Indigenous researchers can identify what works, what does not and why. This empowers Indigenous people to make the best decisions to support their communities and to meet their needs and aspirations. This doesn't stop non-Indigenous researchers from being involved in this research, as long as they follow this best practice in ethical and scientific approaches. It means that the research will be better and is more likely to be relevant, accurate and translatable, as was the case with the cot death and child health survey data described earlier. Aboriginal people (the community reference group, the researchers and community members) should be involved in defining the purpose and nature of the research, planning the project, data collection, data analysis, return of data and results to community via the reference group, with effective dissemination of learnings, results and publications.

After years working in this area, I (Sandra) am a big believer in the role of research in improving the health of Aboriginal people. Yet the gains we have made as a result of research can be taken away by businesses and lobby groups, which have no regard for the wellbeing of individual Aboriginal people and families. Big and powerful food, alcohol and tobacco companies drive changes that provide poor quality food and beverages that have made it remarkably hard for individuals to remain a healthy body weight or avoid substance abuse. These businesses appear to have much more influence with governments in making decisions about how we live than our careful, quality research. Even in my current studies of young people, we are concerned about increased risks for heart disease and diabetes in them and across generations. However, we can never go back to the bad old days when Aboriginal people were absent from the research teams and were largely the objects of white researchers' gaze. More sophisticated measures are required to counter the advertising and advocacy of unhealthy activities promoted by these lobby groups. This is needed to ensure that Aboriginal people are not left behind as new technologies are developed to power and lengthen the lives of those with privilege and power in Australia and elsewhere in the world.

10

PLANETARY HEALTH: ANCIENT WISDOM FOR MODERN PROBLEMS

FIONA STANLEY, SANDRA EADES AND SHAWANA ANDREWS

This series on First Knowledges has described the very different worldviews between Aboriginal and non-Aboriginal people in Australia. The books explain how First Knowledges are still in existence and that, after decades of ignoring them, there is increasing global interest in how they can be used in many areas of our lives. It is an exciting time to work in Aboriginal health, as the power and depth of Indigenous knowledges are now starting to be valued. Evidence is mounting that the best ways to improve Aboriginal people's successful participation in Australian society and support good health are through the marriage of revitalised Aboriginal knowledges with the necessary Western medicine to manage the diseases that First Nations people have faced since colonisation. Aboriginal people need to lead these new, culturally adaptive ways of providing care if these new ways are to succeed. There are also rapidly increasing cohorts of Aboriginal health professionals who have managed to *walk in both worlds,* having the expertise of Western medicine as well as driving the revitalisation of Aboriginal worldviews. Birthing and dying on Country and Aboriginal community-controlled medical services are great examples of this, as is the success with which Aboriginal leadership managed the COVID-19 pandemic.[1]

When Norman Swan[2] interviewed Fiona and Donna Ah Chee about the Voice to Parliament being a health issue, he asked Donna to describe for the listeners what an Aboriginal community-controlled health service was. Donna Ah Chee is CEO of Central Australian Aboriginal Congress, one of the largest and most successful Aboriginal community-controlled organisations in Australia. As she described Congress in Alice Springs, with its holistic approaches and focus on families, Norman commented, 'Well, that is a health service we would all like to have.' He really got it! We feel that the mainstream services in Australia could benefit from Indigenous knowledges in many areas, not just health.

In thinking about health, we have discussed the connectedness of the First Knowledges world, that humans are only a part of a wonderful web of dependent interactions with land, waterways, sky (stars, moon and sun), animals and plants. They are fully entwined in spiritual connections, with stories shared between generations for millennia.

These stories tell of why the world is how it is, how the animals, the stars, the shape of the country and the waterways were created. Passed down orally, they also tell of how we need to live together, with wise kinship systems that ensure populations are genetically robust. The health of people is just a logical result of how this wonderful circular thinking works – from conception to birth to growth through life to death and back to conception again – with laws that ensure participation and conforming. People's health comes from caring for the health of this environment and particularly for Country according to very well-known and strict laws. For 65,000 years this intimate understanding of the land, the seasons and the skies has guided when to move, what to hunt and harvest and what ceremonies to perform. It has been used to ensure that all life on Earth was valued, with the understanding that if you cared for land, it would care for you. This was a clearly sustainable way of living. Sustainable not just for your lifetime, but for those not yet born and coming in future generations.

The remarkable marri (red gum) tree had many medicinal uses (for example, the gum is very effective for injuries and burns). However, its other fascinating use was that its internal trunks had been removed during its growth to create a bowl to catch water. This action, done several generations earlier, was not for those ancestors at all but for the people of today. Is this thoughtful planning for sustainable futures one of the most important lessons that we can learn from First Knowledges? What do these ways of thinking about planetary health and future planning for health and wellbeing mean for us in today's world? A world facing huge environmental and climate catastrophes.

The dominant Western world's structures and worldview are vastly different and have had the opposite effect on the planet than that of Indigenous populations. Indigenous knowledges in other nations such as Canada, the United States and Scandinavia are similarly conservationist and sustainable – First Nations in Canada speak of how what we do now needs to be planned as to how it will affect the next seven generations. The European colonisation of these populations has been based on a culture of hierarchy and dominance, not only of the Indigenous populations but of the land on which they were living. Empires were created from small European countries (England, Spain, Holland, France, etc.) colonising large areas of most of the world (Africa, India, Australia, the Americas, Indonesia and the Pacific Islands). Their hierarchical view of racial superiority was clear – white Europeans at the top and Indigenous populations at the bottom. And contrary to Indigenous worldviews of including land, flora and fauna in one's value systems, these were viewed as needing to be controlled and dominated to exploit the wealth they contained. This capitalist view, so damaging to Australia's Indigenous people, has been catastrophic for our environment and more broadly, for our planet.

Western capitalism's predatory economic systems are based on greed – the push for wealth creation has driven many developed and increasingly developing countries to pursue unfettered growth and increased consumption. Gross Domestic Product (GDP) is used internationally by countries and global organisations (including the World Bank, International Monetary Fund) as *the singular* measure of what makes a successful society. The focus is on increasing wealth without thinking of the damaging effects of how the wealth was created, or how it is used to improve society (or not). This became increasingly popular during the 1980s when Margaret Thatcher, Ronald Reagan and Milton Friedman pushed financial success as the best measure of how a country was performing. Over the last forty years, this capitalism has become more extreme, expanding globally, and is the underlying cause of the disastrous planetary effects observed today.

In Australia, as in all developed countries, this devotion to GDP as our singular measure of societal success has devastated much of our country. Much of the cherished and nurtured lands of Aboriginal peoples who lived here in harmony for thousands of years have been destroyed by these approaches to wealth creation. As well as the negative impacts on Country through the introduction of cattle and sheep, the pastoral industry was built on the slave labour of Aboriginal families who worked for many years receiving only food rations and poor accommodation and facing removal from their traditional lands and ways. The mining and fossil industries have been the most damaging for Indigenous lands and peoples, particularly in those states with large deposits of iron ore, coal, gas, gold and other minerals.

As increasing GDP has become the most powerful and influential driver of all countries, with devastating results for planetary health, it also influences the health and wellbeing of its citizens. Mental-health problems (such as anxiety, depression and substance abuse) have increased, and so has obesity, leading to an increase in diseases such as diabetes, heart disease and strokes.

The costs of services have escalated, and a lack of community trust and feelings of powerlessness are replacing altruism and caring communities.[3] Science and evidence are not just ignored in relation to climate change but in many other areas, such as our health-care systems. These now focus on huge investments in private services that work mainly when disease is inevitable rather than at prevention, which would be more humane and far less costly.

Clearly GDP is not a good measure of societal progress. It counts all economic activity as positive, including many economic activities that reduce wellbeing, such as tobacco, military weapons, guns and pollutants. It ignores non-market production, such as unpaid domestic work and volunteering. Some of the key societal factors that enhance wellbeing, such as health, education, working conditions, equity, time use, social relations and citizenship, are being ignored, as are the factors essential to sustain wellbeing – how we look after our environments for enhancing human and social capacity.

First Nations peoples form the majority of people in many countries who bear the brunt of environmental damage, climate change and the failure and inequities of capitalism. However, in 2023, Indigenous peoples are managing 24 per cent (almost 55,000 million metric tonnes) of the global carbon stored above ground in the world's tropical forests.[4] Despite contributing the least to global environmental changes, Indigenous communities worldwide experience the inequitable impacts of these changes.[5] Many global corporations and wealthy individuals have the most powerful and influential voices in decision making, in many instances over and above any government. They are the ones who stand to gain the most from short-term wealth, while science and evidence are denigrated and ignored, increasing the concerns of our citizens.

As Noel Nannup has said, 'It's like the planet is screaming at the top of its lungs and no one is listening.'[6]

Planetary health has now become an emerging Western concept that *at last* acknowledges that human health is intricately connected to the health of natural systems within the Earth's biosphere and that the health of all species is deeply reliant on it.[7] These understandings have rapidly changed many people's thinking, but our major corporations and many governments do not wish to act, or if they do, it is not quickly enough. They are still too strongly influenced by the wealth creation mantra. We believe that solutions to planetary health can be found in bringing together Indigenous knowledges and innovative science, as we have recommended for health and welfare services. This process needs to come with humility, true sharing of power and knowledge and a sense of urgency and deep commitment from humanity to understand the fragility of our existence. We do need to act – and act now.

Indigenous knowledge systems and values are of great importance to countering the global human catastrophe that is unfolding as a result of the separation of people and nature. Balance with nature, reciprocity and the obligation to help those in need are key principles within Indigenous economies. They promote sufficiency rather than infinite growth, and equity and redistribution of wealth rather than accumulation. Many subsistence economies are also characterised by circular agriculture models, which minimise waste and carbon emissions. The revitalisation, continuation and flourishing of Indigenous knowledges require significant changes in many of the environments and circumstances that continue to undermine them, and which relegate Indigenous people and their wisdom to the sidelines of reform efforts in social, legal, agricultural, environmental, economic and political systems.

Traditional ecological knowledges, from land management to health care, have become subjects of critical interest among experts looking for solutions. Cultural burning, for example, is a practice Aboriginal people use to manage the health of Country.[8] As settlers took over the lands, Aboriginal people no longer had access to their Country to care for it through practices such as cultural burns. However, in recent time there is a growing awareness in mainstream Australia that these burns are an essential way to address the occurrence of extreme bushfires caused by climate change.[9]

The link between the management of Country in this way and health is evident. Across Naarm, for example, she-oak forests and woodlands were made accessible by productive land management. They attracted flocks of emus, mobs of kangaroos, echidnas and a large range of other animals. In the dry summer Kulin season of Biderap, the smell of smoke from ancient fire burning practices, sanctioned by Elders, would hang in the air. The Wurundjeri people used fire to manage the land and to promote new growth, which as well as attracting animals would provide the right conditions for particular tuberous plants to grow, such as myrnong.[10] As a staple food crop across much of southeastern Australia, myrnong was intensely harvested and used as both a nutritious root vegetable and herb. Grazing by introduced stock and exotic pastures marked the rapid decline of the myrnong. Many environmentalists, farmers, bureaucrats and politicians are now seeking the knowledge Elders hold not only about cultural burning but also other agricultural practices. Indigenous ranger programs are being funded around the continent to harness this enduring and sophisticated evidence-based Aboriginal knowledge of Country and its management.

These Indigenous agricultural models are being picked up by Indigenous social enterprises and by organisations such as Parks Australia. One example is Booderee National Park on the New South Wales south coast. Booderee is Aboriginal land for which the Wreck Bay Aboriginal community fought long and hard. Now owned by the Wreck Bay Aboriginal Community Council, the park is jointly managed by Wreck Bay Enterprises – a wholly Indigenous-owned venture established by the council for the socioeconomic benefit of the community – and Parks Australia, 'using a mix of Indigenous knowledge and Western science'.[11] The council plans and manages housing, social welfare, education, training and the health needs of community members; protects and conserves important natural and cultural places; does land use planning; and manages and maintains Aboriginal land. For the Wreck Bay Aboriginal Community, having title to their land has given them the opportunity to be an equal partner in the region's economy.[12]

An exciting recent report, *25 Years of Indigenous Protected Areas*,[13] describes the growth in number and spread of Indigenous Protected Areas in Australia. From five in 1998–99 there are now eighty-four across tropical, desert and temperate ecosystems (87 million hectares of land and 6 million hectares of sea). Run by Traditional Owners and employing Indigenous rangers, they are having a positive impact on conservation, biodiversity and endangered species. They are serving as models for how traditional knowledges can make a significant difference to sustainable land management.

Despite this increasing recognition of traditional knowledges, they have often been applied across the globe in ways that are more symbolic than practical. For example, employing a token Aboriginal Elder to 'advise' on a Western agricultural business is not going to result in that business being helped by traditional knowledge. Employing some Aboriginal health workers in a mainstream health service will not create a service that is culturally safe, unless they have control. Traditional knowledges are not meant to be an assortment of cherry-picked information that can simply be merged with Western scientific knowledge systems.[14] Traditional knowledges are specific to the Country in which each Indigenous language group has expertise. They are collective, holistic, community-based, land-informed ways of knowing that are inherently interconnected with people and the environment. They are applicable in local communities and distinct ecosystems and may be diminished if scaled up, as they depend on local knowledge and historical wisdom that is passed down within a particular community. Ways of burning Country, for example, will differ between Kimberley Country in the north of Western Australia and the forests in the southwest of the state.

However, the *principles* of Indigenous knowledges can be used widely. We have described in earlier chapters the connected ways in which Dreaming stories and Songlines form the basis of knowledge systems such as kinship and understandings of place, and how cultural practice supports this. Work is required to revitalise these knowledges, ensuring they keep their integrity as they are applied anew across the world. Is it too late for mainstream Australia to learn from our Indigenous brothers and sisters to heal our country and reverse the impacts of colonialist capitalism? Can we engage our citizens, encouraging them to vote for solutions such as banning fossil-fuel mining and stopping over-consumption and degradation?

The critical and urgent need for a rethinking of the prevailing economic growth model for mainland Australians is even more urgent for Torres Strait Islanders and Pacific Island nations. The need for approaches that prioritise biodiversity, cultures, Indigenous knowledge and relationships has now been woven into at least five pillars of the Pacific Islands Forum's 2050 Pacific Strategy.[15] The First Nations communities of Australia and Oceania are not only bearing the brunt of carbon capitalism, but they are also leading the fight against it in the courts and elsewhere. In 2022, a group of eight Torres Strait Islander people made legal history when they successfully petitioned the UN Human Rights Committee. The committee found climate change was already affecting the Torres Strait Islander people's daily lives, and that Australia's poor climate record violated the global human rights treaty, the International Covenant on Civil and Political Rights (ICCPR).[16]

This book describes the powerful and effective Indigenous knowledges, for health and for wellbeing; it explores Aboriginal ways of knowing, being and doing that are ancient and sophisticated. They do not need 'modernising', but their applicability requires nuanced and respectful management so they can be of benefit not just to Aboriginal people, but for all of us. We feel strongly that 'reweaving Australia's ecological map needs to be considered not just for health services, but for all ways of living in this country'.[17]

ULURU STATEMENT FROM THE HEART: WHAT IT MEANS FOR FIRST KNOWLEDGES – HEALTH

In words that are beautiful and full of truths, the Uluru Statement from the Heart clearly reflects our thinking and deliberations about First Knowledges. The invitation it gives is for all Australians to share in this knowledge for a better future, if we can walk together. Our strong message is that the solutions to our huge societal challenges, not just health, could come from us walking together.

ULU_RU STATEMENT FROM THE HEART

We, gathered at the 2017 National Constitutional Convention, coming from all points of the southern sky, make this statement from the heart:

Our Aboriginal and Torres Strait Islander tribes were the first sovereign Nations of the Australian continent and its adjacent islands, and possessed it under our own laws and customs. This our ancestors did, according to the reckoning of our culture, from the Creation, according to the common law from 'time immemorial', and according to science more than 60,000 years ago.

This sovereignty is *a spiritual notion: the ancestral tie between the land, or 'mother nature', and the Aboriginal and Torres Strait Islander peoples who were born therefrom, remain attached thereto, and must one day return thither to be united with our ancestors. This link is the basis of the ownership of the soil, or better, of sovereignty.* It has never been ceded or extinguished, and co-exists with the sovereignty of the Crown.

How could it be otherwise? That peoples possessed a land for sixty millennia and this sacred link disappears from world history in merely the last two hundred years?

With substantive constitutional change and structural reform, we believe this ancient sovereignty can shine through as a fuller expression of Australia's nationhood.

Proportionally, we are the most incarcerated people on the planet. We are not an innately criminal people. Our children are aliened from their families at unprecedented rates. This cannot be because we have no love for them. And our youth languish in detention in obscene numbers. They should be our hope for the future.

These dimensions of our crisis tell plainly the structural nature of our problem. This is *the torment of our powerlessness*.

We seek constitutional reforms to empower our people and take *a rightful place* in our own country. When we have power over our destiny our children will flourish. They will walk in two worlds and their culture will be a gift to their country.

We call for the establishment of a First Nations Voice enshrined in the Constitution.

Makarrata is the culmination of our agenda: *the coming together after a struggle*. It captures our aspirations for a fair and truthful relationship with the people of Australia and a better future for our children based on justice and self-determination.

We seek a Makarrata Commission to supervise a process of agreement-making between governments and First Nations and truth-telling about our history.

In 1967 we were counted, in 2017 we seek to be heard. We leave base camp and start our trek across this vast country. We invite you to walk with us in a movement of the Australian people for a better future.

ACKNOWLEDGEMENTS

I would like to acknowledge all those who supported the writing of this book, and in particular the advice and support of Aunty Patsy Cameron, Aunty Lola Greeno, Anne Kennedy, Aunty Dr Sarah Berg, Uncle Jim Berg, David Clarke, Dr Jane Miller, Prof. Glenn Bowes, Yoolongteeyt Aunty Dr Vicki Couzens, Aunty Gina Bundle, Aunty Joy Murphy, Dr Josh Cubillo, Lisa Kennedy, and all those who have shared their knowledge with me over the years and whose work I have cited. –SA

I would like to acknowledge my family, my first teachers who guided my first understanding of the world around me and the values that have carried me through life. My mother Gwen Eades always believed in me and encouraged me in my academic interests and pursuits from an early age. My sister Francine Eades shared University and lifelong work and personal adventures and support along with my other siblings Stafford, Darryl and Tracey. I also acknowledge my late brother Ivan.

I acknowledge Professor Rob Sanson-Fisher an important mentor who shaped and supported my early entry into medicine from school.

At the outset of my research career I was fortunate to meet Fiona Stanley and Anne Read who supervised my PhD, laid solid foundations for my research career and remain lifelong friends.

I would like to acknowledge the early pioneers and leaders in Aboriginal health including Ted Wilkes, Shane Houston and Aunty

Joan Winch. I am grateful for having met and learned from Naomi Myers, Puggy Hunter, Ian Anderson, and to have worked with Shaun Ewen, Shawana Andrews, Robyn Williams, Dan McAullay and my Aunty Anne-Marie Eades. Thank you to my friends and colleagues Emily Banks and Jessica Stewart who provide sage advice and inspiration. –SE

I would like to thank esteemed Noongar Elders, and friends, Millie Penny (also an artist), Fred Penny and Dr Noel Nannup for sharing so generously their wonderful stories and knowledge about Indigenous world views. And heartfelt thanks to Yindjibarndi Elder, Matriarch, artist and friend, Tootsie Daniels for her wisdom and for allowing me to quote her. Dr Marion Kickett (Noongar from York) shared the York Birthing Tree photograph, which is in chapter 3, thank you.

I mention in my personal introduction that I have been privileged to work with an outstanding group of Aboriginal researchers since setting up the Telethon Kids Institute in 1990. We have shared our knowledges, wisdom and experiences in ways that have enriched my life beyond measure. I feel that I am a better person and researcher because of these friendships, which have influenced my thinking so much. They have told me about the daily racism they have faced, the challenges of their early lives that they managed to overcome, and the fight they had to gain their degrees and to be accepted as health professionals.

I list these scholars here in alphabetical order:

Professor Dawn Bessarab, Bard/Yjindjabandi; Professor Ngiare Brown, Yuin NSW; Professor Juli Coffin, Nyangumarta;

ACKNOWLEDGEMENTS

Dr Heather d'Antoine, Gija; Professor Pat Dudgeon, Bardi woman, Kimberley, WA; Professor Sandra Eades, Minang Noongar, WA; Professor Jan Hammill (deceased 2021); Associate Professor Jocelyn Jones, Noongar; Professor Cheryl Kickett-Tucker, Wadjuk Noongar; Associate Professor Glenn Pearson, Noongar; Professor Rhonda Marriott, Nyikina, Kimberley, WA; Professor Helen Milroy, Palyku, Pilbara, WA; Professor Daniel McAullay, Noongar; Professor Ted Wilkes, Noongar; Professor Michael Wright, Yuet Noongar.

Thank you to Christian Crozier, who helped with the references in my chapters.

Associate Professor Deborah Lehmann, Dr Roz Walker and Dr Anne Read are non-Indigenous researchers who were key to the success of our Aboriginal training and research programs. –FS

IMAGE CREDITS

Front inside cover *Replanting the Birth Trees*, 2022

Valerie Ah Chee is a proud Bindjareb woman from the Nyoongar Nation in the southwest of Western Australia, with family connections to the Palyku people of the Pilbara. A proud mother of six and grandmother of six beautiful grandchildren. Valerie is a midwife and comes from a long line of incredibly strong and amazing Nyoongar women who inspire her to try and do her best in everything. Her work is very representative of the strength of women in all aspects of life, especially in pregnancy, birthing and mothering. Valerie is currently working at Stillbirth CRE as an Indigenous Research Midwife, developing strength-based and culturally safe resources and education with the team to reduce the risks of preventable stillbirths in Aboriginal communities.

Back inside cover Yoorrook Justice Commission (2022) The Yoorrook Methodology, developed by Commissioner Sue-Anne Hunter. Artwork by Anjee-Lee Bamblett.

22 BA2750/884: Gwen Eades with her daughter Sandra (detail), Western Australia, ca. 1975.
Photo: Ron Williams
Sourced from the collections of the State Library of Western Australia and reproduced with the permission of the Library Board of Western Australia.

IMAGE CREDITS

64 Professor Marion Kickett, a Ballardong woman from York, Western Australia, with Fiona Stanley in front of one of the birthing trees in York, November 2023. The last traditional birth there was in the 1840s.
Photo: Dr Susan Downes

127 *Reproduction of a Gunditjmara possum skin cloak collected in 1872 from Lake Condah*, 2002 by Debra Couzens and Vicki Couzens, Gunditjmara/Keerray Woorroong people, National Museum of Australia.
© Debra Couzens and Vicki Couzens/Copyright Agency, 2024.

NOTES

INTRODUCTION
1 JM Willis, 'Dying in Country: Implications of culture in the delivery of palliative care in indigenous Australian communities', *Anthropology & Medicine*, 6, 1999, pp. 423–35.
2 A McMichael, *Climate Change and the Health of Nations: Famines, Fevers, and the Fate of Populations*, Oxford University Press, 2017.
3 Marcia Anderson, Ian Anderson, Janet Smylie, Sue Crengle & Mihi Ratima, *Measuring the Health of Aboriginal and Torres Strait Islander Peoples*, Discussion Paper, Onemda VicHealth Koori Health Unit, no. 16, 2006.
4 J Krakouer, 'Wise Counsel Mock Panel', *Gathering the Seeds Symposium Report*, University of Melbourne, Parkville, Victoria, 2 October 2023, p. 27.
5 B O'Dea, Y Roe, Y Gao, S Kruske, C Nelson, S Hickey, A Carson, K Watego, J Currie, R Blackman, M Reynolds, K Wilson, J Costello & S Kildea, 'Breaking the Cycle: Effect of a multi-agency maternity service redesign on reducing the over-representation of Aboriginal and Torres Strait Islander newborns in out-of-home care: A prospective, non-randomised, intervention study in urban Australia', *Child Abuse & Neglect*, 149, 13 February 2024.

2. PLACE, RELATIONSHIPS AND FUTURES
1 Ian Anderson, 'On the Passing of Dr Yunupingu AM (1948–2023)', *Pearls and Irritations: John Menadue's Public Policy Journal*, 5 April 2023.
2 Dr Yunupiŋu, 'Rom Watangu', *The Monthly*, 1 July 2016.
3 Binmila Yunupiŋu, 'Yunupiŋu Family Statement', Yothu Yindi Foundation, 3 April 2023, <gy.yyf.com.au/#family_statement>.
4 Bruce Pascoe & Bill Gammage, *Country: Future Fire, Future Farming*, First Knowledges series, Thames & Hudson Australia, 2021.
5 Media release, 'Western Australia's 27,000 year old mine announced for National Heritage Listing', Yamatji Marlpa Aboriginal Corporation, 25 February 2011. See also: Government of Western Australia, 'Ochre',

State Library of Western Australia website: Mining & Energy WA, 2 September 2023, <exhibitions.slwa.wa.gov.au/s/mewa/page/ochre>.
6   Carlos M Duarte, 'Red ochre and shells: clues to human evolution', *Trends in ecology & evolution*, 29(10), 2014, pp. 560–65.
7   Joseph Velo, 'Ochre as medicine: a suggestion for the interpretation of the archaeological record', *Current Anthropology*, 25(5), 1984, pp. 674–74.
8   Jillian Huntley, 'Australian Indigenous ochres: Use, sourcing, and exchange', in I McNiven, B David (eds), *The Oxford Handbook of the Archaeology of Indigenous Australia and New Guinea*, Oxford University Press, 2021.
9   Marcia Langton & Aaron Corn, *Law: The Way of the Ancestors*, First Knowledges series, Thames & Hudson Australia, 2023.
10 Patricia Cameron, 'Grease and ochre: the blending of two cultures at the Tasmanian colonial sea frontier', Masters thesis, University of Tasmania, 2008, p. 42.
11 Janice Reid, *Sorcerers and Healing Spirits*, Australian National University Press, Canberra, 1983.
12 Anthony Rex Peile, *Body and Soul: An Aboriginal view*, Aboriginal Studies Series no. 10. Hesperian Press, 1997.
13 Ngaanyatjarra, Pitjantjatjara & Yankunytjatjara, Women's Council Aboriginal Corporation, *Traditional Healers of Central Australia: Ngangkari*, Magabala Books, Broome, 2013.
14 *Traditional Healers of Central Australia*, 2013.
15 Marcia Anderson, Ian Anderson, Janet Smylie, Sue Crengle & Mihi Ratima, *Measuring the Health of Aboriginal and Torres Strait Islander Peoples*, Discussion Paper, Onemda VicHealth Koori Health Unit, no. 16, 2006.
16 Gija People, 'Jirraginy joo Goorrarndal: Frog and Brolga' animation, Sharing Stories Foundation website, <sharingstoriesfoundation.org/resource/jirraginy-joo-goorrarndal-frog-and-brolga-animation/>.
17 National Aboriginal Health Strategy Working Party, *A National Aboriginal Health Strategy*. NAHS Working Party, Canberra, 1989.
18 Kaiela Institute, 'Dungala Kaiela Oration', Kaiela Institute website, <kaielainstitute.org.au/dungala-kaiela-oration.html>.

3. BIRTHING ON COUNTRY AND DYING ON COUNTRY

1 Aunty Tootsie Daniels, Personal communication with the author, 2023.
2 J Smylie, M Kirst, K McShane, M Firestone, S Wolfe, P O'Campo, 'Understanding the role of Indigenous community participation in Indigenous prenatal and infant–toddler health promotion programs in Canada: A realist review', *Social Science & Medicine*, 150, February 2016, pp. 128–43.
3 M Lyon, M Aboutalebi Karkavandi, D Cameron, R Gayde, P Gray, H Milroy, C Davison and C Chamberlain for the 'Replanting the Birthing Trees' Investigators and Project Team. *Gathering the Seeds Symposium Report*, University of Melbourne, Parkville, Victoria, 2 October 2023.
4 Y Roe, 'Birthing Healthy and Strong Babies on Country', *Medical Research Future Fund Report*, Australian Government, Department of Health and Aged Care website, May 2023.
5 S Henry, 'Koori Maternity Services', *Obstetrics & Gynaecology Magazine*, 25(1), 2023.
6 AC Parry, 'Boodjari Yorga's Midwifery Group Practice', in *Gathering the Seeds Symposium Report*, University of Melbourne, Parkville, Victoria, 2 October 2023, p. 26.
7 Professor Rhonda Marriott, lead researcher, 'Birthing on Noongar Boodjar project', Ngangk Yira Institute for Change, Murdoch University, 9 March 2023.
8 Valerie Ah Chee, text printed on a card that was one of the *Gathering the Seeds* Symposium handouts, 2023.
9 S Henry, 'Koori Maternity Services', *Obstetrics & Gynaecology Magazine*, 25(1), 2023.
10 L Nelson, 'The Importance of the Right Support for Families', *Gathering the Seeds Symposium Report*, University of Melbourne, Parkville, Victoria, 2 October 2023, p. 21.
11 AC Parry, 'Boodjari Yorga's Midwifery Group Practice', *Gathering the Seeds Symposium Report*, University of Melbourne, Parkville, Victoria, 2 October 2023, p. 26.
12 E Carter, J Lumley, G Wilson, S Bell, '"Alukura ... for my daughters and their daughters and their daughters", A review of Congress Alukura',

Australian and New Zealand Journal of Public Health, 28(3), June 2004, pp. 229–34.

13 S Kildea, S Hickey, L Barclay, et al., 'Implementing Birthing on Country services for Aboriginal and Torres Strait Islander families: RISE Framework', *Women Birth*, October 2019, 32(5), pp. 466–75.

14 S Cousins, 'Birthing on Country: Improving maternal care in Australia', *The Lancet*, 21 January 2023, 401(10372), pp. 184–85.

15 P McCalman, D Forster, T Springall, M Newton, F McLardie-Hore & H McLachlan, 'Exploring satisfaction among women having a First Nations baby at one of three maternity hospitals offering culturally specific continuity of midwife care in Victoria, Australia: A cross-sectional survey', *Women Birth*, 36(6), Nov 2023.

16 P McCalman, D Forster, T Springall, M Newton, F McLardie-Hore & H McLachlan, *Women Birth*, 36(6), November 2023.

17 S Ireland, Y Roe, S Moore, S Kildea, et al., 'Birthing on Country for the best start in life: Returning childbirth services to Yolŋu mothers, babies and communities in North East Arnhem, Northern Territory', *Medical Journal of Australia*, 217(1), 4 July 2022, pp. 5–8.

18 S Cousins, *The Lancet*, 21 January 2023, 401(10372), pp. 184–85.

19 J Krakouer, 'Wise Counsel Mock Panel', *Gathering the Seeds Symposium Report*, University of Melbourne, Parkville, Victoria, 2 October 2023, p. 27.

20 B O'Dea, Y Roe, Y Gao, S Kruske, C Nelson, S Hickey, A Carson, K Watego, J Currie, R Blackman, M Reynolds, K Wilson, J Costello & S Kildea, 'Breaking the Cycle: Effect of a multi-agency maternity service redesign on reducing the over-representation of Aboriginal and Torres Strait Islander newborns in out-of-home care: A prospective, non-randomised, intervention study in urban Australia', *Child Abuse & Neglect*, 149, 13 February 2024.

21 AC Parry, 'Boodjari Yorga's Midwifery Group Practice', *Gathering the Seeds Symposium Report*, University of Melbourne, Parkville, Victoria, 2 October 2023, p. 26.

22 P McCalman, D Forster, T Springall, M Newton, F McLardie-Hore & H McLachlan, *Women Birth*, 36(6), Nov 2023.

23 Baby Coming You Ready?, <babycomingyouready.org.au>.

24 SMS4Dads, <www.sms4dads.com.au>.
25 R Owen, M Miller, *Placenta Garden and Ceremony: Cultural Revival for Wellbeing*, Wathaurong Aboriginal Cooperative.
26 Jill Gallagher quoted in R Owen, M Miller, Wathaurong Aboriginal Cooperative.
27 D Nelson, R Marriott, T Reibel, *Ngangk Waangening: Mothers' Stories*, Ngangk Yira Research Centre for Aboriginal Health and Social Equity, 2021.
28 L Nelson, 'The Importance of the Right Support for Families', *Gathering the Seeds Symposium Report*, University of Melbourne, Parkville, Victoria, 2 October 2023, p. 21.
29 JM Willis, 'Dying in Country: Implications of culture in the delivery of palliative care in indigenous Australian communities', *Anthropology & Medicine*, 6, 1999, pp. 423–35.
30 D Wake, J Dineen, K Martin, 'Yarlparu: On sorrow. Talking to the families of dying Aboriginal people', *Australian Nursing Journal*, 6, 1 April 1999.
31 D Wake, J Dineen, K Martin, *Australian Nursing Journal*, 6(9), 1 April 1999.
32 D Wake, J Dineen, K Martin, *Australian Nursing Journal*, 6(9), 1 April 1999.
33 JM Willis, *Anthropology & Medicine*, 6, 1999, pp. 423–35.
34 Corporation WDNWPTA, Purple House, <purplehouse.org.au/>.
35 Corporation WDNWPTA, Purple House.
36 JM Willis, *Anthropology & Medicine*, 6, 1999, pp. 423–35.
37 P McGrath, E Phillips, 'Insights on end-of-life ceremonial practices of Australian Aboriginal peoples', *Collegian*, 15(4), 2008, pp. 125–33.

4. COMMUNITY CONTROL AND PRIMARY HEALTH CARE

1 A Haebich, 'Aboriginal Assimilation and Nyungar Health 1948–72', *Health and History*, 14(2), 2012, pp. 140–61.
2 D P Thomas, *Reading Doctors' Writing: Race, Politics and Power in Indigenous Health Research, 1870–1969*, Aboriginal Studies Press for the Australian Institute of Aboriginal and Torres Strait Islander Studies, Canberra, 2004.

3 L Youngsub & K Gyoungsup, 'The Turning Point of China's Rural Public Health during the Cultural Revolution Period: Barefoot Doctors: A Narrative', *Iranian Journal of Public Health*, 47, 2018, pp. 1–8.
4 Australian Government, *A National Aboriginal Health Strategy 1989*, 2023, <webarchive.nla.gov.au/awa/20090918180530/http://www.health.gov.au/internet/main/publishing.nsf/Content/health-oatsih-pubs-NAHS1998>.
5 Australian Government, *A National Aboriginal Health Strategy 1989*.
6 Australian Government, *A National Aboriginal Health Strategy 1989*, 2023; definition quoted from Declaration of Alma-Ata, International Conference on Primary Health Care, Alma-Ata, USSR, 6–12 September 1978.
7 Katharine Viner, 'More than $500m to be cut from Indigenous programs in Budget', *The Guardian*, 13 May 2014.
8 NACCHO, *National Aboriginal Community Controlled Health Organisation: Our Story*, 2023, <naccho.org.au/our-story/>.
9 DYHS, *Derbarl Yerrigan Health Service Annual Report 2022/2023*, 2023.
10 C Bower, et al., 'Fetal alcohol spectrum disorder and youth justice: a prevalence study among young people sentenced to detention in Western Australia', *BMJ Open*, 8(2), 2018, p. e019605.

5. INDIGENOUS PEOPLE AND HOSPITAL CARE

1 Ronald D Wilson & Meredith Wilkie, *Bringing Them Home: Report of the National Inquiry into the Separation of Aboriginal and Torres Strait Islander Children from their Families*, Human Rights and Equal Opportunity Commission, Sydney, Australia, 1997.
2 Irihapeti Ramsden, *Cultural safety and nursing education in Aotearoa and Te Waipounamu*, Dissertation, Victoria University of Wellington, 2002.
3 Patrick Wolfe, 'Settler Colonialism and the Elimination of the Native', *Journal of Genocide Research*, 8(4), 2006, pp. 387–409.
4 Commonwealth of Australia, 'Aboriginal welfare, conference of Commonwealth and State Ministers, Commonwealth Parliamentary Papers', vol. iii, 19623, Darwin, July 1963, p. 651.
5 Ian Wronski, 'The Growth and Development of under-5 Aboriginal Children in Shepparton and Mooroopna', Health Commission of Victoria, 1980.

6 Angela Clarke, Shawana Andrews & Neville Austin, *Lookin' after our own: Supporting Aboriginal families through the hospital experience*, Victorian Health Promotion Foundation, Aboriginal Family Support Unit, Royal Children's Hospital, 1999.

7 Clarke, et al., Victorian Health Promotion Foundation, Aboriginal Family Support Unit, Royal Children's Hospital, 1999.

8 Ian Anderson, 'Koorie health in Koorie hands: An orientation manual in Aboriginal health for health-care providers', Koorie Health Unit, Health Department, Victoria, 1988.

9 Note VAHS was the second ACCHO, Redfern was the first in 1971.

10 Clarke, et al., Victorian Health Promotion Foundation, Aboriginal Family Support Unit, Royal Children's Hospital, 1999.

11 Dr Sarah Berg, personal communication with the author, 15 November 2023.

12 Lina Gubhaju, Robyn Williams, Jocelyn Jones, David Hamer, Carrington Shepherd, Dan McAullay, Sandra J Eades & Bridgette McNamara, '"Cultural security is an on-going journey ..." Exploring views from staff members on the quality and cultural security of services for Aboriginal families in Western Australia', *International Journal of Environmental Research and Public Health*, 17(22), 2020, p. 8480.

13 Now called the Australian Human Rights Commission.

14 Patricia Dudgeon & Abigail Bray, 'Indigenous relationality: Women, kinship and the law', *Genealogy* 3, 2(23), 2019, p. 2.

15 Clarke, et al., Victorian Health Promotion Foundation, Aboriginal Family Support Unit, Royal Children's Hospital, 1999.

16 Clarke, et al., Victorian Health Promotion Foundation, Aboriginal Family Support Unit, Royal Children's Hospital, 1999, p. 64.

17 Kathryn Priest, Sharijn King, Wendy Nungurrayi Brown, Irene Nangala & Marilyn Nangala, 'Warrki Jarrinjaku, "Working together everyone and listening": Growing together as leaders for Aboriginal children in remote central Australia', *European Early Childhood Education Research Journal*, 16(1), 2008.

18 C Chamberlain, S Andrews, M Langton, et al., 'Supporting Aboriginal and Torres Strait Islander Families to Stay Together from the Start (SAFeST Start): Urgent call to action to address crisis

in infant removals', *Australian Journal of Social Issues*, 57(2), 2022, pp. 252–73.

19 Clarke, et al., Victorian Health Promotion Foundation, Aboriginal Family Support Unit, Royal Children's Hospital, 1999.

20 Margaret A Kelaher, Angeline S Ferdinand & Yin Paradies, 'Experiencing racism in health care: The mental health impacts for Victorian Aboriginal communities', *Medical Journal of Australia*, 201(1), 2014, pp. 44–7.

6. TRADITIONAL LIFE FOR HEALTH

1 M Arnold, *A journey travelled: Aboriginal-European relations at Albany and the surrounding region from first contact to 1926*, UWA Publishing, Crawley, Western Australia, 2015.

2 J Host and C Owen, *'It's still in my heart, this is my country': The Single Noongar Claim History*, UWA Publishing, Crawley, WA, 2020, 2009.

3 V Hansen and J Horsfall, *Noongar Bush Medicine: Medicinal plants of the south-west of Western Australia*, UWA Publishing, Crawley, WA, 2020, 2016.

4 B R Maslin, *WATTLE: Acacias of Australia*, 2018, <apps.lucidcentral.org/wattle/text/entities/acacia_microbotrya.htm>.

5 V Hansen and J Horsfall, *Noongar Bush Tucker: Bush food plants and fungi of the south-west of Western Australia*, UWA Publishing, Crawley, Western Australia, 2019.

6 V Hansen and J Horsfall, UWA Publishing, Crawley, Western Australia, 2019.

7 G L Curtis, et al., 'Impact of Physical Activity in Cardiovascular and Musculoskeletal Health: Can Motion Be Medicine?', *Journal of Clinical Medicine Research*, 2017, 9(5), pp. 375–81.

8 P A Coventry, et al., 'Nature-based outdoor activities for mental and physical health: Systematic review and meta-analysis', *SSM – Population Health*, 2021, 16, p. 100934.

9 K O'Dea, 'Marked improvement in carbohydrate and lipid metabolism in diabetic Australian Aborigines after temporary reversion to traditional lifestyle', *Diabetes*, 1984, 33(6), pp. 596–603.

10 P C Hallal, et al., 'Physical activity: more of the same is not enough', *The Lancet*, 2012, 380, pp. 190–91.

7. HEALTH AND CULTURAL PRACTICE

1 Yothu Yindi Foundation, August 2023.
2 J Liddle, M Langton, JWW Rose & Simon Rice, 'New thinking about old ways: Cultural continuity for improved mental health of young Central Australian Aboriginal men', *Early Intervention in Psychiatry*, 16(4), 24 June 2021, pp. 461–65.
3 Shawana Andrews, 'Cloaked in Strength: How possum skin cloaking can support Aboriginal women's voice in family violence research', *AlterNative: An International Journal of Indigenous Peoples*, 16(2), 2020, pp. 108–16.
4 Michael J Chandler & Christopher E Lalonde, 'Cultural continuity as a protective factor against suicide in First Nations youth', *Horizons*, 10(1), 2008, pp. 68–72.
5 Michael J Chandler & Christopher E Lalonde, 'Cultural continuity as a hedge against suicide in Canada's First Nations', *Transcultural psychiatry*, 35(2), 1998, pp. 191–219.
6 Joseph P Gone, 'Redressing First Nations historical trauma: Theorizing mechanisms for Indigenous culture as mental health treatment', *Transcultural Psychiatry*, 50(5), 2013, pp. 683–706.
7 Margo Rowan, Nancy Poole, Beverley Shea, Joseph P Gone, David Mykota, Marwa Farag, Carol Hopkins, Laura Hall, Christopher Mushquash & Colleen Dell, 'Cultural interventions to treat addictions in Indigenous populations: Findings from a scoping study', *Substance abuse treatment, prevention, and policy*, 9(1), 2014, pp. 1–27.
8 J Liddle et al., *Early Intervention in Psychiatry*, 16(4), 24 June 2021, pp. 461–65.
9 Lola Greeno, 'Retracing the History of the Tasmanian Aboriginal Shell Necklaces', *Ponrabble*, 23 February 2020, <ponrabbel.blogspot.com/2020/02/retracing-history-of-tasmanian.html>.
10 NJB Plomley, *A word-list of the Tasmanian Aboriginal languages*, The State of Tasmania, 1976, pp. 279 & 472.

11 Shawana Andrews & Aunty Patsy Cameron, Personal communication, 4 September 2023.
12 Shawana Andrews & Aunty Patsy Cameron, Personal communication, 4 September 2023.
13 Aunty Joy Murphy, illustrated by Lisa Kennedy, *Welcome to Country*, Walker Books Australia, NSW, 2016.
14 Benjamin Mabo, 'Languages Alive', Australian Institute of Aboriginal and Torres Strait Islander Studies, 24 March 2023, <aiatsis.gov.au/explore/languages-alive>.
15 Andrew Butcher, 'Linguistic aspects of Australian Aboriginal English', *Clinical linguistics & phonetics*, 22(8), 2008, pp. 625–42.
16 Greg Dickson, 'Explainer: The largest language spoken exclusively in Australia – Kriol', *The Conversation*, 26 April 2016.
17 Aunty Patsy Cameron, *Grease and ochre: The blending of two cultures at the colonial sea frontier*. Fullers Bookshop, 2011.
18 George Augustus Robinson, *Friendly mission: the Tasmanian journals and papers of George Augustus Robinson, 1829–1834*, Queen Victoria Museum and Art Gallery, 2008.
19 Michelle K H K Gantevoort, 'Stingray in the sky: Astronomy in Tasmanian Aboriginal Culture and Heritage', Honours Thesis, University of New South Wales, 2015.
20 Eva McRae-Williams, John Guenther, Damien Jacobsen & Judith Lovell, 'What are the enablers of economic participation in remote and very remote Australia, and how can we identify them?', *Learning Communities: International Journal of Learning in Social Contexts*, vol. n/a, no. 19, 2016, pp. 6–25.
21 Bruce Pascoe, *Dark Emu: Aboriginal Australia and the birth of agriculture*, Magabala Books, 2018, p. 71.
22 B Pascoe, Magabala Books, 2018, p. 206.
23 Department of Climate Change, Energy, the Environment and Water, 'National Heritage Places: Mount William Stone Hatchet Quarry', Australian Government, 25 February 2008, <dcceew.gov.au/parks-heritage/heritage/places/national/mount-william>.
24 Adam Brumm, '"The Falling Sky": Symbolic and Cosmological Associations of the Mt William Greenstone Axe Quarry, Central

Victoria, Australia', *Cambridge Archaeological Journal*, Cambridge University Press, 20(2), pp. 179–96, 2010.
25 A Brumm, 20(2), *Cambridge Archaeological Journal*, pp. 179–96, 2010.
26 A Brumm, 20(2), *Cambridge Archaeological Journal*.

8. ABORIGINAL WORLDVIEWS IN MAINSTREAM SERVICES

1 *Ngurra warndurala buluyugayi: Exploring Yindjibarndi country*, Juluwarlu Aboriginal Corporation, Roebourne, Western Australia, 2007.
2 M Wright, T Culbong, M Webb, et al., 'Debakarn Koorliny Wangkiny: Steady walking and talking using First Nations-led participatory action research methodologies to build relationships', *Health Sociology Review*, 13 March 2023, pp. 1–18.
3 M Wright, A Lin, & M O'Connell, 'Humility, inquisitiveness, and openness: Key attributes for meaningful engagement with Nyoongar people', *Advances in Mental Health*, 14, 2016, pp. 82–95.
4 M Wright, T Culbong, M Webb, et al., *Health Sociology Review*, 13 March 2023, pp. 1–18.
5 Author's personal correspondence with M Wright.
6 M Wright, T Culbong, M Webb, et al., *Health Sociology Review*, 13 March 2023, pp. 1–18.
7 M Wright, T Culbong, M Webb, et al., *Health Sociology Review*, 13 March 2023, pp. 1–18.
8 Australian Government, *Bringing Them Home* Report (1997): Report of the National Inquiry into the Separation of Aboriginal and Torres Strait Islander Children from their Families, Australian Human Rights Commission, 1997.
9 S Hamilton, *Critical Capital: Recovery and Justice*, ANU College of Law, 2023.
10 S Hamilton, 2023.
11 S Hamilton, 2023.
12 S Hamilton, 2023.
13 SL Hamilton, S Maslen, B Farrant, N Ilich, C Michie, '"We don't want you to come in and make a decision for us": Traversing cultural authority and responsive regulation in Australian child protection systems', *Australian Journal of Social Issues*, 57(2), 2022, pp. 236–51.

14 C Liddle, CEO of SNAICC, *Family Matters Report 2022: Measuring trends to turn the tide on the over-representation of Aboriginal and Torres Strait Islander children in out-of-home care in Australia*, 2022, <familymatters.org.au>.
15 S Hamilton, 2023.
16 Figure 1, F Stanley, adapted from 'Historical impacts of colonisation upon Indigenous health', J D Mathews, 'The Menzies School of Health Research offers a new paradigm of cooperative research, Medical Research Perspectives', *Medical Journal of Australia*, 169 (11), 14 December 1998.
17 H Davidson, 'Child protection cases more than doubled after NT Intervention, inquiry told', *The Guardian*, 19 June 2017.
18 Christine Andre Jeffries-Stokes, *Goolleelar Ngoodah!: A qualitative study of the attitudes of the Aboriginal people of the Eastern Goldfields of Western Australia to the health services offered to them and comparison with the perceptions of the medical staff providing those services*, Master of Public Health thesis, University of Western Australia, Dept of Public Health, 1996.
19 ABC *Four Corners*, 'Heart Failure: An investigation into the hidden killer in remote Australian communities', Australian Broadcasting Corporation, 2022, 45:17 minutes.
20 Productivity Commission, *Closing the Gap Annual Data Compilation Report*, July 2023.
21 F Stanley, M Langton, J Ward, D McAullay, S Eades, 'Australian First Nations response to the pandemic: A dramatic reversal of the "gap"', *Journal of Paediatrics and Child Health*, 57(12), December 2021, pp. 1853–56.
22 ABC *Health Report*, 'Why The Voice is a health issue', Australian Broadcasting Corporation, 2023.

9. AN INDIGENOUS-LED HEALTH RESEARCH AGENDA
1 R Bainbridge, K Tsey, J McCalman, et al., 'No one's discussing the elephant in the room: Contemplating questions of research impact and benefit in Aboriginal and Torres Strait Islander Australian health research', *BMC Public Health*, 15(1), 23 July 2015, p. 696.

2 DP Thomas, R Bainbridge, K Tsey, 'Changing discourses in Aboriginal and Torres Strait Islander health research, 1914–2014', *Medical Journal of Australia*, 201(1 Suppl), 7 July 2014, S15–18.

3 JF Seward, FJ Stanley, 'Comparison of births to Aboriginal and Caucasian mothers in Western Australia', *Medical Journal of Australia*, 25 July 1981, 2(2), pp. 80–84.

4 Productivity Commission, *Closing the Gap Annual Data Compilation Report July 2021*.

5 SJ Eades, *Bibbulung Gnarneep (Solid Kid) : A longitudinal study of a population based cohort of urban Aboriginal children in Western Australia: Determinants of health outcomes during early childhood of Aboriginal children residing in an urban area*. PhD Thesis, University of Western Australia, 2004.

6 National Aboriginal Health Strategy Working Party, *A National Aboriginal Health Strategy*, NAHSW, Canberra, 1989.

7 S J Eades, 'The RAWG Research Roadmap Background Paper: Maternal health, infancy, childhood and adolescent focused research, laying the foundation for a lifetime of health for ATSI people', NHMRC, Canberra, 2001.

8 S J Eades, AW Read, 'The Bibbulung Gnarneep Project: Practical implementation of guidelines on ethics in indigenous health research', *Medical Journal of Australia*, 170(9), 3 May 1999, pp. 433–36.

9 A D'Aprano, C Lloyd-Johnsen, D Cameron, et al., 'Trusting relationships and learning together: A rapid review of Indigenous reference groups in Australian Indigenous health research', *Australian and New Zealand Journal of Public Health*, 47(3), June 2023, p. 100051.

10 D Bessarab, B Ng'andu, 'Yarning about yarning as a legitimate method in Indigenous research', *International Journal of Critical Indigenous Studies*, 23(1), 2010, pp. 37–50.

11 For more information see: ' WA Aboriginal Child Health Survey (WAACHS)', Telethon Kids Institute website, www.telethonkids.org.au/our-research/Indigenous-health/waachs/

12 S Silburn, S Zubrick, D Lawrence, F Mitrou, J DeMaio, E Blair, et al., 'The intergenerational effects of forced separation on the social and

emotional wellbeing of Aboriginal children and young people', *Family Matters*, 75, 2006, pp. 10–17.
13. ABC *Four Corners*, 'Backing Bourke', Australian Broadcasting Corporation, 2016.
14. *Justice Reinvestment in Bourke* Briefing Paper, Australian Human Rigths Commission, Aboriginal Legal Service, Just Reinvent, NSW, 2013.
15. T Kukutai, J Taylor (eds), *Indigenous Data Sovereignty: Toward An Agenda*, ANU Press, Canberra, 2016.
16. United Nations Declaration on the Rights of Indigenous Peoples (UNDRIP), United Nations, 2007.
17. *Indigenous Data Sovereignty Communique*, Indigenous Data Sovereignty Summit, Maiam nayri Wingara Indigenous Data Sovereignty Collective and the Australian Indigenous Governance Institute, Canberra, ACT, 20 June 2018. For articles about data sovereignity see also: Lowitja Institute website, www.lowitja.org.au/?s=data+sovereignty+.

10. PLANETARY HEALTH: ANCIENT WISDOM FOR MODERN PROBLEMS

1. F Stanley, M Langton, J Ward, D McAullay, S Eades, 'Australian First Nations response to the pandemic: A dramatic reversal of the 'gap'', *Journal of Paediatrics and Child Health*, 57(12), December 2021, pp. 1853–56.
2. *ABC Health Report*, 'Why The Voice is a health issue', Australian Broadcasting Corporation, 2023.
3. K Lycett, F Stanley, 'The Health and Wellbeing of Future Generations', chapter in E Dawson, J McCalman, *What Happens Next: Reconstruction Australia after COVID-19*, Melbourne University Press, 2020.
4. DE Mamo, *The Indigenous World 2020*, 34th ed., The International Working Group for Indigenous Affairs (IWGIA), Copenhagen, Denmark, 2020.
5. N Redvers, Y Celidwen, C Schultz, et al., 'The determinants of planetary health: an Indigenous consensus perspective', *Lancet Planet Health*, 6(2), February 2022, e156–e163.
6. Noel Nannup, Noongar Elder, personal communication with FS, 2023.
7. A McMichael, *Climate Change and the Health of Nations: Famines, Fevers, and the Fate of Populations*, Oxford University Press, 2017.

8   B Gammage, B Pascoe, *Country: Future Fire, Future Farming,* First Knowledges series, Thames & Hudson Australia, 2021.
9   See 'What is cultural burning', Australian Musuem website, <https://australian.museum/learn/teachers/classroom-activities/cultural-burning/>.
10 N Zola, B Gott, *Koorie plants, Koorie people: Traditional Aboriginal food, fibre and healing plants of Victoria*, Koorie Heritage Trust, Melbourne, 1992.
11 See <parksaustralia.gov.au/booderee/>.
12 R Colbourne, 'Indigenous Entrepreneurship and Hybrid Ventures', in A Corbett, J Katz (eds), *Perspectives & Approaches to Blended Value Entrepreneurship*, volume 19, 'Advances in Entrepreneurship, Firm Emergence and Growth', Emerald Publishing.
13 *25 Years of Indigenous Protected Areas: Keeping Country Strong,* Country Needs People , 2023, <www.countryneedspeople.org.au/25-years-of-ipas>.
14 M Ratima, D Martin, H Castleden, T Delormier, 'Indigenous voices and knowledge systems: Promoting planetary health, health equity, and sustainable development now and for future generations', *Global Health Promotion,* 26(3 suppl), April 2019, pp. 3–5.
15 *2050 Strategy for the Blue Pacific Continent*, Pacific Islands Forum Secretariat, Suva, Fiji, 2022.
16 C Bird, R Monson, 'Australia's Climate Neglect on trial in the Torres Strait Islands', *The Saturday Paper,* 24–30 June 2023.
17 C Bird, R Monson, *The Saturday Paper,* 24–30 June 2023.

FURTHER READING

Cameron, Aunty Patsy, illustrated by Lisa Kennedy, *Sea Country* (Magabala Books, Broome, WA, 2021).

Chamberlin, J. Edward, *If this is Your Land, Where are Your Stories?*, Vintage, Canada, 2004.

Clarke, Angela, Shawana Andrews & Neville Austin, *Lookin' after our own: Supporting Aboriginal families through the hospital experience* (Victorian Health Promotion Foundation, Aboriginal Family Support Unit, Royal Children's Hospital, 1999).

David, B, R Mullett, N Wright, et al., 'Archaeological evidence of an ethnographically documented Australian Aboriginal ritual dated to the last ice age'. *Nature Human Behaviour* (1 July 2024). <https://doi.org/10.1038/s41562-024-01912-w>.

Dodson, Patrick, Hal Wootten, Daniel O'Dea, Lew Wyvill, Elliott Johnston, *Royal Commission into Aboriginal Deaths in Custody: Final Report* (Royal Commission into Aboriginal Deaths in Custody, Government of Australia, 15 April 1991).

Eckermann, Ali Cobby, *She is the Earth*, Magabala Books, 2023.

Gay'wu Group of Women, *Songspirals: Sharing women's wisdom of Country through songlines*, Allen & Unwin, 2019.

Hansen, Vivienne & John Horsfall, *Noongar Bush Tucker: Bush food plants and fungi of the south-west of Western Australia* (UWA Publishing, WA, 2019.

Hansen, Vivienne & John Horsfall, *Noongar Bush Medicine: Medicinal Plants of south-west of Western Australia* (UWA Publishing, Crawley, WA, 2016).

Harjo, Joy, 'Perhaps the World Ends Here' in *The Woman Who Fell From the Sky* (W. W. Norton and Company Inc., 1994).

Jones, Ross L, James Waghorne, Marcia Langton, *Dhoombak Goobgoowana: A History of Indigenous Australia and the University of Melbourne. Volume 1: Truth*, MUP, 2024.

Kickett-Tucker, C, D Bessarab, J Coffin & M Wright (eds), *Mia Mia Aboriginal Community Development: Fostering Cultural Security* (Cambridge University Press, Melbourne, 2017).

King, Madison & John Horsfall, *Bush Medicine: Medicinal plants of the Kimberley Region of Western Australian* (UWA Publishing, Crawley, WA, 2023).

Kowal, Emma, *Haunting Biology: Science and Indigeneity in Australia (Experimental Futures)* (Duke University Press, USA, 2023).

Langton, Marcia, *Welcome to Country*, 2nd edition (Hardie Grant Explore, Melbourne, 2021).

Murphy, Aunty Joy, illustrated by Lisa Kennedy, *Welcome to Country* (Walker Books Australia, NSW, 2016).

Murphy, Aunty Joy, illustrated by Lisa Kennedy, *Wilam: A Birrarung Story*, (Walker Books Australia, NSW, 2019).

O'Connor, Emily, et at., 'He Ara Waiora/A Pathway towards Wellbeing', Discussion Paper, 20 September 2018, NZ Treasury.

Quilliam, Wayne, *Culture is Life*, Hardie Grant Publishing, 2021.

Rintoul, Stuart, *Lowitja: The authorised biography of Lowitja O'Donoghue* (Allen & Unwin, NSW, 2020).

Yoorook For Justice: Report into Victoria's Child Protection and Criminal Justice System (Yoorook Justice Commission, Melbourne, 2023).

INDEX

Note: Page numbers in **bold** refer to captions or images.

25 Years of Indigenous Protected Areas, 183

Aaniiih-Gros Ventre tribal nation (US), 128
Abbott, Tony, 85
ABC, 168–9
Aboriginal Advancement Council, East Perth, 30, 78
Aboriginal Community-Controlled Health Services, 78
Aboriginal Community Participation Action Research, 8, 33, 142–3, 147, 156, 165, 173
Aboriginal English, 133
Aboriginal Family Support Unit, RCHM, 99, 101, 103, 106
Aboriginal healers, *see* traditional healers
Aboriginal health services, 78–80, 87–9
Aboriginal health systems, 6–7, 42–4, 82–3, 93
Aboriginal health workers, 32, 78–80, 170, 184
Aboriginal Hospital Liaison Officers, 94–6, 98, 106
Aboriginal knowledge, *see* traditional knowledge
Aboriginal Liaison Policy Advisory Committee, 98
Aboriginal Medical Service Congress (1986), 54
Aboriginal Medical Service, Redfern, 46, 78, 81
Aboriginal parenting practices, 97, 105
Aboriginal worldviews, and mainstream health services, 141–50, 176
ADHD, 88
agriculture, 136
Ah Chee, Donna, 176
Ah Chee, Valerie, 51–2
Albany, 108–9, 116
Anangu people, 69
Ancestral Beings, 44–5, 68, 134
Anderson, Ian, 163–4
antacids, 38
antenatal care, 56, 170
antiseptics, 3, 38
Aotearoa, 172
Apology to the Stolen Generations (2008), 85–6
aquaculture, 136
Arnhem Land, 3, 15–16, 67–8, 123
assimilation, 75–8, 93, 105
astronomy, 6
Australian Bureau of Statistics, 172

INDEX

Australian Indigenous Governance Institute, 172
Australian National University, 80
Australian native medicines, viii, 2
axe stone, 137

Baby Coming You Ready? (digital platform), 59
'barefoot doctor' program, 79–80
Barunga Statement, 35
Bates, Daisy, 77
Batman Treaty, 137
Beejenup, 115
Bellear, Lisa, 18
Berg, Sarah, 95
Biderap, 182
Billibellary, 137
Birak, 110–11
birds, 116
birthing: Aboriginal women in mainstream hospitals, 57–9; Birthing on Country movement, 54–9, 63; birthing support programs, 52–3, 59, 62–3; Grandmothers' Way of birthing, 9, 51–2, 54–6; in Western health systems, 57–8; infections in pregnancy, 169–70; on Country, 9–10, 49–63, 72, 176; on missions and reserves, 73–4; preterm births, 55, 57, 169
Birthing on Noongar Boodjar Project, 51, 62
Birthing on Noongar Boodjar–Nhangk Waagening, 62
birthing trees, 60–1, **64**, 141
Black Power movement, 31

Black War, 130
blood samples, 171
bogong moths, 18
Booderee National Park, New South Wales, 183
Boodjari Moort/Kwilenap, 63
Boodjari Yorgas, 51, 53
Boorloo (Perth), 24
Bourke, 168–9
breastfeeding, 55, 170
Briggs, Dalrymple, 19
Bringing Them Home Report, 85, 91, 96, 147
brolgas, 44
Broomehill, 115
Bubup Wilam, 153
Bulla Meeyle, 114
Bulman-Weemol community, 16
Bundle, Gina, 126
Bunuru, 110–13
Buŋgal, 123
burns, 38
Burrup Peninsula, 50
bush medicine, 2, 41
bush saunas, 3

Cameron, Patsy, 40, 130, 133
Canada, 178
cancer, 22–3, 27, 66
Cape Barren goose, 38–9
capitalism, 178–80
carbon storage, 180
Carter, Emily, 152
Carter, Maureen, 152
Central Australia, 69
Central Australian Aboriginal Congress, 46, 176
Central Desert, 67–8

ceremony, 129
cervical cancer screening, 88
Chamberlain, Cath, 51
Chandler, Michael J, 126–7
Charles Darwin University, 54
Chief Protector of Aborigines, 76
Child and Parent Centre, Fitzroy Valley, 152
child mortality, 57
Child Protection, 103–4, 147
children: Aboriginal child-rearing practices, 97, 105; Aboriginal children in hospital, 90–1, 97–8, 102–4; child care, 152–3; developmental problems, 88–9; infant vaccination, 170; removal of from families, 29, 85–6, 91, 93, 96, 147, 149; sexual abuse of, 154
China, 79–80
chitty chitty (willy wagtails), 116
Christianity, 70
chuck-a-luck (wattlebirds), 116
citizenship, for Indigenous Australians, 75
Clarke, Angela, 91–2, 95, 98–9, 101, 103, 106–7
cleansing ceremonies, 2, 68
climate change, 180, 185
Closing the Gap, 85–6, 152, 155
Co-operative Research Centre in Aboriginal and Tropical Health, 164
Coalition government, 153
Coalition of Peaks, 86, 89
coastal pigface, 112
Coastal Plains Nation, 38, 40–1, 134–5

colonisation: Aboriginal health prior to, 39; based on hierarchy and dominance, 178; decolonising the management of First Nations people, 143–4; effect on cultural identity, 126; impact on Indigenous people, 46, 76, 93, 109, 150–2, **151**, 159, 161; in Trouwerner, 131; strategy of dismantling Aboriginal culture, 132
community control, of health services, 84, 89, 142, 176
community health nurses, 25–6
community participation, 8–10, 78, 154, 168–9
Community Reference Groups, 173
community trust, erosion of, 180
Congress Alukura, Alice Springs, 54
consent, in hospitals, 101–2
Cook, James, 5–6
Coolbaroo League, The, 77
Coombs, Kevin, 94
Coppin, Lorraine, 140–1
Corn, Aaron, 6
cot deaths, 165–6
Country: birthing on, 9–10, 49–63, 72, 176; defined, 36–7; dying on, 9–10, 28, 50, 64–72, 176; in Aboriginal economies, 135; in the National Aboriginal Health Strategy, 82; managing health of, 182; personal perspectives on, 19–20, 23; primacy of, 1–2; relation to health, 5, 36, 177; *see also* place
Couzens, Debra, **127**

Couzens, Yoolongteeyt Vicki, 125, **127**
COVID-19 pandemic, 10, 69, 89, 176
Cranbrook, 21–2, 111
crayfish, 38
crying rooms, 7
cultural burning, 182–4
cultural dynamism, 155
cultural identity, 126–7
cultural practices, and health, 123–38
Cultural Revolution, China, 79–80

dance, 123–4
Daniels, Tootsie, 49–50
Dark Emu (Pascoe), 136
data collection, *see* Indigenous data collection
data sovereignty, *see* Indigenous data sovereignty
death: Aboriginal conception of, 2; attending to sorry business, 4, 70–1; dying on Country, 9–10, 28, 50, 64–72, 176; in the Noongar world view, 66; mortuary practices, 28, 67–8, 70–1; personal perspectives of, 22–4, 27–9; respect for Aboriginal protocols, 5, 7, 43
'death rain', 23
Debakarn Koorliny Wangkiny, 142
dental care, 53
Derbal Yerrigan (formerly Perth Aboriginal Medical Service), 32, 87–9, 162
developmental problems, in children, 88–9
diabetes, 118–19, 179

dialysis, 50, 68–9
diarrhoea, 2, 38
diet, 39, 117–19
disease, introduction of, 93
Djeren, 110, 113
Djilba, 110, 116
Dodson, Mick, 96
domestic violence support, 53, 63
Dreaming, 134, 184
ducks, 114
Dunbar, Terry, 164
Dungala Kaiela Oration, 47

Eades, Gwen, **22**
Eades, Howard, 77
Eades, Sidney, 77, 79, 111, 115
Eades, Stafford, 75, 115
ear disease, 170
early childhood programs, 169–70
Eastern Goldfields, 169–70
economic growth, 178–81
economics, and health, 135–8, 178–82
Elders, 105, 126, 141, 143–50, 165–7, 183–4
Elston, Jacinta, 164
emu, 116
environmental change, 180
epidemiological studies, 161–2
epilepsy, 23
European worldview, 149–50
evidence-based studies, 180
exercise, 3–4, 110, 117–18, 120–1

FASD, 88
fetal alcohol syndrome, 88, 152

firestick burning, 111, 182–4
First Knowledges series, 1–13, 175
First Nation support rooms, 7
fish weirs, 110
fishing, 110–11
Flinders Island, 38, 130
flowers, 117
Flying Doctor, 29–30
food, 1–2, 38–41, 140, 182–3; *see also* diet; nutrition
fossil fuel industry, 179
Four Corners (television program), 168
Friedman, Milton, 179
Frontier Wars, 93
funerals, 70–1
Furneaux Islands, 130
futures (stories), 44–8

Gallagher, Jill, 61–2
Garma Festival, 123–4
Gathering the Seeds Symposium, 50–3, 63, 71
Gemini constellation, 134
gender, 40–1
Geraldton Hospital, 66
Gija Country, 44–5
Giles, 29
gilgies, 112
Gnowangerup mission, 73–5
goanna oil, 28
Gone, Joseph, 128–9
Gorogo, Danielle, ii, **ii**
Gove Land Rights case, 34
Grandmothers' Way, of birthing, 9, 51–2, 54–6, 98
grandparents, 105

greed, 178–9
green ants, 3
Greeno, Lola, 129
greenstone quarry, 137–8
Gross Domestic Product, 178–80
The Growth and Development of under 5 Aboriginal Children in Shepparton and Mooroopna (Wronski), 94
Gulkula, 123
gum trees, 112, 177
Gumatj clan, 34, 123
Gunaikurnai people, 17
Gunditjmara Country, 44
Gunditjmara people, 100, **127**
Gunditjmara possum skin cloak, **127**
Gundjarraŋbuy, Rosemary, 53

Haebich, Anna, 75–7
Half Caste Act, 93
Hamilton, Sharynne, 147–8
Harjo, Joy, 20
Hayward, Denis, 25–6
healers, *see* traditional healers
health: Aboriginal and Western medicine compared, 6–7, 42–4, 82–3; Aboriginal distrust in mainstream services, 154–5; Aboriginal health services, 78–80, 87–9; Aboriginal health systems, 6–7, 42–4, 82–3, 93; Aboriginal health workers, 32, 78–80, 170, 184; Aboriginal worldviews in mainstream health services, 141–50; access to mainstream services, 75–6, 93–4; before colonisation, 39; community control of health

services, 84, 89, 142, 176; cultural safety in provision of services, 91–2, 98–9, 146; defined, 46, 83; impact of colonisation on, 150–2, **151**; planetary health, 176–86; poor conditions on missions and reserves, 73–7; reasons for failure to close the gap, 152; relation to Country, 5, 36, 177; relation to cultural practices, 123–38; relation to economics, 135–8, 178–82; relation to traditional knowledge, 141–50; self-determination in health care, 75–8, 83–4; through traditional life, 108–22; *see also* children; health research

health centres, as community centres, 46

Health Commission of Victoria, 94

health promotion programs, 166

health research: Aboriginal Community Participation Action Research, 8, 33, 142–3, 147, 156, 165, 173; by non-Indigenous people, 157–61, 174; exploitation of by business and lobby groups, 174; Indigenous-led health research, 161–74; mainstream versus Aboriginal, 142–3; research into cot deaths, 165–6; role of the National Health and Medical Research Council, 33, 160–5; strengths-based approach to, 161–5; Western Australia Aboriginal Child Health Survey, 167–8

heart disease, 179

hepatitis C, 88

High Court of Australia, 85

Hockey, Joe, 85

Homelands movement, 3

homelessness, 103

hookworm, 76

hospitals, 90–107; Aboriginal Hospital Liaison Officers, 94–6, 98, 106; 'failure to attend', 103–5; framework for cultural safety, 91–2, 98–9; giving consent, 101–2; respect for Aboriginal practices, 4–5, 65–6, 97–100, 106; *see also specific hospitals*

Houston, Shane, 81, 164

Howard, John, 86

Human Rights and Equal Opportunity Commission, 91

hunter-gatherer lifestyle, 119

India, 18–19

Indigenous data collection, 8–9, 159, 165–70, 172–3

Indigenous data governance, 171, 173

Indigenous data sovereignty, 8–9, 159, 169–74

Indigenous Data Sovereignty Communique, 172–3

Indigenous Protected Areas, 183–4

Indigenous rangers, 183–4

Indigenous Voice to Parliament, 35, 156

infant vaccination, 170

intellectual disabilities, 88–9

intellectual property rights, 2

International Covenant on Civil and Political Rights, 185

International Decade of Indigenous Languages 2022–2032, 133
International Monetary Fund, 178
The Intervention, 8, 154

Jackson, Moana, 47
James Cook University, 164
Jigalong, 29
Juluwarlu Aboriginal Corporation, 140–1

Kalgoorlie, 169
Kambarang, 110, 117
kaolin, 2, 38
Keating, Paul, 85
Keerray people, 125, **127**
Kennedy, Lisa, 124
kick bush, 116
Kickett, Marion, **64**
Kildea, Sue, 54–6
killer whales, 136–7
Kimberley, 184
Kimberley Aboriginal Medical Service, 88
King George Sound, 110
King, Tommy, 76, 109
Kinjarling, 109
kinship systems, 4, 40, 97, 101–2, 105, 131, 148, 184
kitchen table, 20–1
knowledge, *see* traditional knowledge
koolbardies (magpies), 116
koomal, 116
Koori Maternity Service, 51, 53, 55, 60
Koori people, 92

Koorie Health Unit, 94–5
Kriol, 133
Krishnan, Raji, 25
Kulin people, 125, 182
Kulunga, 32

Lalonde, Christopher E, 126–7
The Lancet, 56
land management, 182
land rights, 34, 85, 109
Langton, Marcia, 6, 51
language: existing and endangered languages, 133; language barriers, 101; loss of, 132; not recorded by Australian Bureau of Statistics, 172; relation to cultural identity, 127
Latrobe, 19
Law, 6, 135
Little Children are Sacred Report, 154
Little Mussleroe Bay, 20, 131
logical family, 4
London School of Hygiene and Tropical Medicine, 31
Lookin' After Our Own, 106
Looking Forward Project, 143, 145–6
low-fat diet, 119

Mabo, Eddie, 85
Maiam nayri Wingara Indigenous Data Sovereignty Collective, 172
Makarrata, 189
Makaru, 110, 113–16
Mannalargenna, 19, 38, 134

mapanpa, 41
Marninwarntikura Women's Resource Centre, 152–3
Marr Mooditj, 32, 79–80
Marriott, Rhonda, 51
massacres, 64, 93
maternal mortality, 57
McGrath, Pam, 71
McKenzie, Queenie, 140
measles, 76
media, 161–2, 168–9
medicinal plants, viii, 140
Meekatharra, 66
mental health, 4, 41–2, 118, 179
mental illness, 143, 146
Menzies, Robert, 76
midwives, 55–6, 74
mining industry, 179
missions, 73–5, 93
moieties, 40
Molly Wardaguga Research Centre, 54
mortuary practices, 28, 67–8, 70–1
Mount Barker, 21–2
Mount Barker Hospital, 75
Mount Barker Native Reserve, 74–5
mountain pygmy possum, 18
mourning, 70–1
Mowanjum people, 119
mulls, 116
Murphy, Joy, 124, 132
Murujuga Country, 49
mushrooms, 113
muttonbirds, 38–9
Myers, Naomi, 81
myrnong, 182–3

Naarm (Melbourne), 15, 20, 128, 182
NACCHO, 9, 84–6, 89
naming taboo, 68
Nannup, Noel, 150, 181
National Aboriginal and Islander Health Organisation, 85
National Aboriginal Community Controlled Health Organisation, 9, 84–6, 89
National Aboriginal Health Strategy (1989), 45–7, 81–4
National Aboriginal Health Strategy Working Group, 45, 81, 83
National Health and Medical Research Council, 33, 160–5
National Health and Medical Research Council Research Agenda Working Group, 163
National Health and Medical Research Council Research Roadmaps, 81, 163–4
National Inquiry into the Separation of Aboriginal and Torres Strait Islander Children from their Families (1995-97), 91, 96
native reserves, 21–2, 73–5
native title, 122
nature, effect on mental health, 118
Nelson, Lesley, 63
Nelson, Robynne, 98
Neville, AO, 76
New Era Aboriginal Fellowship, 30, 78, 87
Ngaanyatjarra, Pitjantjatjara and Yankunytjatjara (NPY) Lands, 41–2

Ngaanyatjarra, Pitjantjatjara and Yankunytjatjara Women's Council Aboriginal Corporation, 42
Ngangk Yira Institute for Change, 62
Ngangkari healers, 7, 41–2, 68, 70, 106
Ngank Waangening Project, 62
Ngullak Koolunga Ngullak Koori (Our Children Our Heart), 147
Ngunytju Tjitji Pirni – NTP – mothers, grandmothers all together, 169–70
Ningulabul, 137
Noongar Ballardong Yuet Country, 150
Noongar Country, 24
Noongar language, 32, 87
Noongar Native Title settlement, 122
Noongar people, 26, 62–4, 66, 74–9, 108–17, 121, 143–50, 162
Noonuccal people, 18
Northern Territory Emergency Response, 8, 154
Nullagine, 29
nurses and nurses' aids, 25–6, 29–30
nutrition, 1, 53

obesity, 108, 179
ochre, 37–8
O'Dea, Kerin, 118–20, 164
O'Donohue, Lowita, vii
Onemda, 95
organ transplants, 43–4
Oscar, June, 152
outdoors, and mental health, 118
ownership, concept of, 132

Pacific Islands Forum 2050 Pacific Strategy, 185
Pairrebeenne people, 15, 129–30
Palawa people, 34
palliative care, 27, 65, 68–9, 71, 126
Parkerville Children's Home, 29
Parks Australia, 183
Pascoe, Bruce, 136
Paul, David, 25
Pell, Charmaine, 147
Penny, Fred, 50, 64–7
Penny, Millie, 50, 64, 66–7, 147
'Perhaps the World Ends Here' (Harjo), 20
Perth, 87–8
Perth Aboriginal Medical Service (later Derbarl Yerrigan), 25–6, 30, 32, 79, 81, 87–9, 162
Perth Children's Hospital, 30–1
petroglyphs, 50
Phillips, Emma, 71
physical activity, *see* exercise
Pinjarra, 64, 67
Pinjarra massacre, 64
place, 36–9
placenta gardens, 60–2, 71
planetary health, 176–86
plants, as medicines, viii, 41
Plato, 120
policy, *see* National Aboriginal Health Strategy (1989)
Port Hedland Hospital, 29–30
possum skin cloaks, 7, 106, 125–6, **127**

possums, 116
poverty, 121
pregnancy, *see* birthing
preterm births, 55, 57, 169
primary care, 80, 83–4, 86, 93
protocols, 129
Pullyit, 114
Purdie, Shirley, 140
Purple House, 69–70
Purple Truck, 69

racism, 31, 57, 73–4, 76, 94, 106, 122, 145, 151–2, 178
Ramsden, Irihapeti, 91
Read, Anne, 27, 165
Reagan, Ronald, 179
recreation clubs, 122
red ochre, 2–3, 37
Redfern Speech, 85
referendum (1967), 75
regulation, of Indigenous Australians, 76–7
regulatory theory, 149
relationality, 100, 131–2
relationships, 39–44, 46
remote communities, 30, 68–9, 102
Replanting the Birthing Trees research project, 51
research, *see* health research
respiratory failure, 71
Returned Soldiers League, 77
rheumatic heart disease, 155
ritual, 129
Robinson, George Augustus, 134
Roe, Yvette, 54–6
Roebourne, 140

Royal Children's Hospital Grand Round, 96–7
Royal Children's Hospital, Melbourne, 90–2, 95–9, 104, 106
Royal Commission into Aboriginal Deaths in Custody (1987), 85, 96
Royal Melbourne Hospital, 5, 7
Royal Perth Hospital, 24
Royal Tour (1954), 29
Rudd, Kevin, 85
Rumbalara Football and Netball Club, 122

Sanson-Fisher, Robert, 26
Sasakawa Award, 80
Scandinavia, 178
Schultz, Rosalie, 169
science, 134, 180
seasons, for the Noongar people, 109–17
Secretariat for National Aboriginal and Islander Child Care, 152
segregation, 73–5, 93–4
self-determination, in health care, 75–8, 83–4
Sharing Knowledge (Gorogo), **ii**
shell necklaces, 129–31
Shepparton, 122
short-tailed shearwater, 39
skin group system, 4
Sky Country, 134
Smith, Linda Tuhiwai, 9
smoking ceremonies, 2, 7–8, 68, 106
smoking, support to stop, 53, 121–2
SMS4Dads (website), 59
Snowy River, 17–18
song, 123–4

Songlines, 124, 184
sorry business, 4, 70–1
South West Aboriginal Medical Service (SWAMS), 63, 88
spiritual world, 37, 40, 42, 50, 68, 100, 114, 133, 136, 176–7
sports clubs, 122
Springs, Florence, 25
Standard Australian English, 133
stars, reading of, 133–4
STDs, 88
stereotypes, of Aboriginal people, 145, 161
Stirling, James, 64
Stirling Ranges, 109
Stokes, Geoffrey, 140
Stolen Generations, 29, 85–6, 93, 96, 147, 161, 167
strokes, 179
Strongyloidiasis, 16
substance abuse support, 63, 128–9
Sudden Infant Death Syndrome, 165–6
suicide, 127, 143
sustainable living, 177
SWAMS Boodjari Moort/Kwilenap, 53
Swan, Norman, 176
Sydney Harbour Bridge Reconciliation Walk, 86

Tebrahunna Country, 20, 38
technology, 59
Telethon Kids Institute, 9, 140, 165, 167
tertiary care, 92–3, 106
Thatcher, Margaret, 179

Thomas, David, 76
Thorne, Shirley, 166
Thorpe, Lisa, 152
Thuwarri Thaa, 37
Timbery, Joe, 29
tobacco smoking, 53, 121–2
Toolbroonup, 109, 114
Torres Strait Islanders, 185
totems, 40, 49, 68
traditional healers, 7, 22–3, 41–2, 68, 70, 106
Traditional Healers of Central Australia: Ngangkari, 42
traditional knowledge, 124, 139–50, 178, 181–2, 184–5
traditional life, as a healthy life, 108–22
Trawlwoolway people, 15, 129–30
Trouwerner (Tasmania), 19–20, 38–9, 129–31, 133–5
trust, in mainstream services, 154–5
truth-telling, 145
tuberculosis, 75
Turtle Island, Canada, 19

Uluṟu Statement from the Heart, 187–9
United Nations, 133
United Nations Human Rights Committee, 185
United States, 178
University of Melbourne, 95, 169

vaccinations, 170
VicHealth Koori Health Research Unit, 95

Victorian Aboriginal Community Controlled Health Organisation, 61
Victorian Aboriginal Health Service, 46, 95, 98
Victorian Treaty possum skin cloak, 126
Vinnicombe, Pat, 140
visiting, of friends and family, 19
Voice to Parliament, 35, 156

WA Aboriginal Legal Service, 30, 78
WACOSS Community Service Award, 89
waitch (emu), 116
walking, 115
wallabies, 38
Walley, Pam, 64
Walmajarri language, 152
Wandinyilmernong, 109
Wardaguga, Molly, 54
Warmun people, 140
Wathaurong people, 60–1
Wathaurong Women's Tranquillity Garden, 60–1
wealth creation, 178–81
weight gain, 108
weight loss, 119
Welcome to Country (Murphy), 124, 132
Weld Ranges, Western Australia, 37
welfare services, reluctance to use, 147–8
Western Australia Aboriginal Child Health Survey, 167–8
Western Australia Health Department, 75
Western health systems: Aboriginal and Western medicine compared, 6–7, 42–4, 82–3; Aboriginal worldviews in mainstream health services, 141–50, 176; advice on dying, 66; biomedical construction of health, 6, 42; birthing, 57–8; lack of appreciation of Aboriginal practices, 65; negotiating the constraints of, 9; prevention of access for Aboriginal people, 93
Whadjuk Noongar people, 24
Wil-im-ee Moor-ring, 137
Wilam: A Birrarung Story (Murphy), 124
wild potatoes, 115–16
Wilgie Mia, 37
Wilkes, Ted, 32, 81
Wilson, Sir Ronald, 85, 96
Winch, Joan, 25–6, 79–80
Wingellina, 29
Wittenoom, 30
Woiwurrung language, 132
women, in food production, 40–1
women's knowledge, 130–1
Woodley Michael, 140–1
Woorroong people, **127**
Woretemoeteyenner, 19
World Bank, 178
World Health Organisation, 80
Wreck Bay Aboriginal community, 183
Wreck Bay Enterprises, 183
Wright, Michael, 142–3
Wronski, Ian, 94
Wungening Aboriginal Corporation, 87–8

Wurundjeri Country, 34, 132, 137
Wurundjeri people, 182
Wurundjeri Woi Wurrung Cultural Heritage Aboriginal Corporation, 137

yarning, 166–7
Year 12 retention rates, 10, 153, 162
Yindjibarndi people, 49, 141
Yirrkala Bark Petitions, 34
Yolŋu people, 60, 123–4
yonga, 114–16
Yorgum Healing Services, 87
Yorta Yorta Country, 47
Yuin people, 136–7
Yunupiŋu, Galarrwuy, vii, 34–5

ABOUT THE AUTHORS

Associate Professor Shawana Andrews, PhD is a Pairrebeenne/Trawlwoolway woman of the Tasmanian Coastal Plains Nation. She is Director of the Poche Centre for Indigenous Health and Associate Dean (Indigenous) in the Faculty of Medicine, Dentistry and Health Sciences at The University of Melbourne. Shawana worked for many years in the hospital system as a social worker before qualifying as a public health educator and researcher and moving to higher education. Her work focuses on Aboriginal health, Aboriginal mothering practices and family violence, cultural practice-based methodologies and Aboriginal doctoral advancement and leadership. Shawana is also an artist exploring the connection between women's lived experience and Country.

Professor Sandra Eades, PhD, AO, FASSA, FAHMS, FTSE is a Noongar woman from Mount Barker, Western Australia. She completed her medical degree in 1990 and after working as a GP, started her career in health research at the Telethon Kids Institute. In 2003 she became Australia's first Aboriginal medical doctor to be awarded a PhD. Her PhD investigated the causal pathways and determinants of health among Aboriginal infants in the first year of life. Professor Eades was named NSW Woman of the Year 2006 in recognition of her research contributions to Aboriginal communities and has received a 'Deadly Award' (National Aboriginal and Torres Strait Islander Awards) for Outstanding Achievement in Health. As well as Deputy Dean (Indigenous) in the Faculty of Medicine,

Dentistry and Health Sciences at The University of Melbourne, she is a Professor at the Centre for Epidemiology and Biostatistics, Melbourne School of Population and Global Health.

Professor Fiona Stanley, AC, FAA, FASSA, FAHMS is the Founding Director and Patron of Telethon Kids Institute, a unique multidisciplinary independent research institute focusing on the causes and prevention of major problems affecting children and youth. She is also Distinguished Research Professor, UWA; Hon Professorial Fellow, The University of Melbourne; UNICEF Ambassador for early childhood; Scientific Advisor Doctors for the Environment. Professor Stanley trained overseas in Epidemiology and Maternal and Child Health, established population data sets in Western Australia, including registers of major childhood problems, championed record linkage, and pioneered First Nations leadership in research. She was instrumental in establishing the Australian Research Alliance for Children and Youth, to lobby nationally for investing in children and families for a better society. For her research on behalf of Australia's children and Aboriginal social justice, Professor Stanley was named Australian of the Year in 2003.

The best of both worlds

TITLES IN THE
FIRST KNOWLEDGES SERIES

SONGLINES
Margo Ngawa Neale & Lynne Kelly
(2020)

DESIGN
Alison Page & Paul Memmott
(2021)

COUNTRY
Bill Gammage & Bruce Pascoe
(2021)

ASTRONOMY
Karlie Noon & Krystal De Napoli
(2022)

PLANTS
Zena Cumpston, Michael-Shawn Fletcher & Lesley Head
(2022)

LAW
Marcia Langton & Aaron Corn
(2023)

INNOVATION
Ian J McNiven & Lynette Russell
(2023)

HEALTH
Shawana Andrews, Sandra Eades & Fiona Stanley
(2024)

CEREMONY
Wesley Enoch & Georgia Curran
(2025)

Published in conjunction with the National Museum of Australia
and supported by the Australia Council for the Arts.

Praise for the First Knowledges series ...

'This beautiful, important series is a gift and a tool. Use it well.'
—Tara June Winch

'An in-depth understanding of Indigenous expertise and achievement.'
—Quentin Bryce, AD, CVO, FAAL, FASSA

'Australians are yearning for a different approach to land management. Let this series begin the discussion. Let us allow the discussion to develop and deepen.'
—Bruce Pascoe

'These First Knowledges books are proving among the most fascinating and important titles I have ever read; an astounding gift of wisdom delivered with generosity and optimism, offering no less than a new vision of what Australia is, and what it can be ... they deserve to change minds, lives, and hopefully the development of Australia itself.'
—Jez Ford